RIDING
WITH THE
ROCKETMEN

JAMES WITTS

RIDING WITH THE ROCKETMEN

One Man's Journey on the Shoulders of Cycling Giants

BLOOMSBURY SPORT
LONDON · OXFORD · NEW YORK · NEW DELHI · SYDNEY

BLOOMSBURY SPORT
Bloomsbury Publishing Plc
50 Bedford Square, London, WC1B 3DP, UK
29 Earlsfort Terrace, Dublin 2, Ireland

BLOOMSBURY, BLOOMSBURY SPORT and the Diana logo are trademarks of
Bloomsbury Publishing Plc

First published in Great Britain 2023
Text copyright © James Witts, 2023

A catalogue record for this book is available from the British Library

Library of Congress Cataloguing-in-Publication data has been applied for

ISBN: TPB: 978-1-3994-0350-4; eBook: 978-1-3994-0349-8;
ePDF: 978-1-3994-0351-1

2 4 6 8 10 9 7 5 3 1

Typeset in Minion Pro by Deanta Global Publishing Services, Chennai, India
Printed and bound in Great Britain by CPI Group (UK) Ltd., Croydon, CR0 4YY

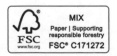

To find out more about our authors and books visit www.bloomsbury.com and sign
up for our newsletters

*To my wife, Tara. You are obviously a pain
but forever 'Rings of Saturn'.*

CONTENTS

PROLOGUE

My name is James Robert Witts. I'm 45 years old and I write about cycling, for magazines, online and the occasional book. I follow the professionals, many of whom are 25 years my junior. That makes me feel old. As do two children who are no longer children. It was only yesterday that I was stick thin and muscles were if not clearly defined, at least perceptible from close range. Now, time and calories have begun to take their toll. I wasn't obese but I have been heading in the wrong direction in recent years. At the end of 2021, I realised that I needed a challenge. 'What about completing a stage of the Tour de France?' no one said to me. 'And what about combining it with your day job by uncovering the secrets of the professionals and then applying similar or watered-down techniques – I'm thinking altitude training, aerodynamic advice, weight-cutting nutrition, rest days… – to my ageing body?' as, again, no one said to me. 'And what about if, in an equally diluted fashion, you complete similar events to the pros along the way?' again, said no one but me. 'You're on,' I said to myself.

And so, in January 2022, began my no-pro journey. The goal event? L'Étape du Tour de France on Saturday 10 July 2022, the Tour de France stage that about 16,000 recreational cyclists have the opportunity to race every year several days before the pros fly past. Confession: it had been sold out for months but one of my freelance roles involves editing the official Tour de France Guide every year, so I took advantage of my privileged position and bagged a media place. Ahead would be 167km of cycling, of which 4700m was climbing, including three of the most famous, and infamous, climbs in Tour de France history: Col du Galibier, Croix de Fer and Alpe d'Huez. I cycle, but not long distances. I've done endurance events in the past – triathlons up to Olympic-distance (1.5km swim, 40km bike, 10km run), a couple of marathons, a few sportives, half-marathons – but few in my

40s and nothing of the magnitude of a long, hot, mountainous day in France. So, there are clearly some obstacles ahead.

In fact, six months of them, to be precise. To mimic the pros would require a level of detail I'd never before applied to my own training. My current fitness levels would need to be assessed, bike position analysed, diet laughed at, training plan set up, build-up events pencilled in, flights planned, accommodation booked … even on paper, it looks tiring. In practice, well, the mind boggles. Then again, my role as a sports hack means I have enviable access to the support teams behind the likes of two-time Tour de France winner Tadej Pogačar, and arguably the finest all-rounder of current times Wout van Aert. Surely, their learnings will inspire me to my own Tour greatness. I mean, how hard could climbing the equivalent of halfway up Mount Everest in one day really be…?

1

The Eye-opener

T-minus seven months until race day

I ride. A reasonable amount. But beyond the occasional mountain-bike session, it's more about commutes that are less than four miles and rack up a single-digit hit in altitude. They're fine for clearing the head and blowing away those sleepy cobwebs; they are not the grounding for the 30th edition of L'Étape du Tour that forums are discussing – and rejoicing over (hardcore cyclists are sadists and take great pleasure in suffering) – as the hardest ever.

On signing up to L'Étape du Tour, I do three things: clean my bike, weigh myself and ride. Or the good, the bad and the ugly. My grime-filled bike is the cleanest it's been for years; I'm 92kg, the highest I've ever been; and my ride out and back from Bristol to the Somerset coastal town of Portishead is cold, wet and windy. It's a 30-mile round trip and I feel more fatigued than I should, especially considering I refuelled on turnaround at one of the many cafes that line Portishead's sparkling new marina.

Still, great oaks from little acorns grow and all that. And with six months ahead to forge myself into a cyclist that'll surely have Sir Dave Brailsford knocking at my door, I have time on my side. And I'll have the knowledge, too. I've spent my career interviewing the world's finest cycling cyclists, from Peter Sagan in Gran Canaria, to Tao Geoghegan Hart in Mallorca and Sir Bradley Wiggins in … Portsmouth. My contacts book of recent times is far more detailed and denser than my training diary. I might lament the long hours, but sports writing has afforded me the fortunate position of holding a direct line to the world's best riders and, arguably more important for my own travails, the world's best cycling coaches, exercise physiologists and sports nutritionists.

That's why there's a template that I'll follow (hopefully) all the way to that finish line at the peak of Alpe d'Huez on Saturday 10 July 2022, in both my training journey and this book. In each chapter, the first half will explore what makes the pro cycling peloton tick, uncovering the extraordinary leaps in science that have made it all (legally) possible. I'll then take these learnings, apply the ones that are realistic for someone with a full-time job and a mid-40s body, and seek further specific one-on-one advice from experts who spend more time with recreational folk like me than the world's svelte and speedy elite. The latter makes up the second half of each chapter; in other words, it's the ideal married to realism.

To that end, we start with the world's finest, followed by me, myself and I. Whatever happens, it's going to be one hell of a journey...

December into the start of January is professional road cycling's off-season, a time for reflection, resolutions and riding. This is when the world's finest cyclists shift into gear for the upcoming race season, seeking warmth, mountainous terrain and smooth roads. Cycling teams such as Ineos Grenadiers head to Mallorca, Trek–Segafredo to Sierra Nevada, and Bora–Hansgrohe to Grenada for camps that are essentially an all-over audit. Here, sports scientists fitness test the riders, coaches prescribe training plans based on a catalogue of physiological data and nutritionists check riders' body fat, even though to the naked eye levels are so low that you can see every vein, artery and sinew under the skin.

It's all in the name of marrying nature with nurture, of ensuring a happy and long-lasting unity before the seasonal passage of time depletes power output, lung capacity and endurance. And what better place to lay the foundations for any marriage than that bastion of monogamy, Benidorm. It's an incongruous backdrop to the world's most monastic sports stars, but within its hedonistic shadows nestles Dénia, where UAE Team Emirates and their talisman Tadej Pogačar are hosting their January training camp

I'm meant to be there to watch and learn, to see just how the Slovenian and his teammates recalibrate and reset for another brutal season, where July's Tour de France is the goal event. Sadly, however, the winter of 2021/2022 was blasted by the tail end of the Covid tornado. Twenty-four hours after booking my flight to Alicante, the team's press officer pulled down the shutters on media attendance. 'Under orders from the team doctors, the media-day interviews will now be moved to a virtual event,' the team's public face, Luke Maguire, informed me. 'Contact won't be allowed, unfortunately.'

And so began a mid-winter cha-cha-cha of acceptance, booking and cancellation followed by Zoom meetings. The (metaphorical) dance of disappointment reprised memories of a brief (and literal) stint salsa dancing with my wife. My wife has rhythm and is never happier than strutting her stuff to disco; rhythm and I have never been formally introduced and I'm at my most unsettled when within dragging distance of a dance floor. I've forever protested that males over 1.8m should be banned from dancing, unless you're Massive Attack's Daddy G, who possesses astonishing dexterity for someone of 1.96m. Mind you, salsa briefly coaxed out some unique moves and I began to enjoy tapping my feet to the timing of the beat during classes, until I fell off my bike and broke my ankle, which brought my dancing days to an abrupt halt. Even though I recovered, I saw it as a sign that cycling didn't want me to be the next Revel Horwood and I never side-stepped again.

I don't know whether George Bennett is a great dancer but I suspect not as he's 1.8m tall on the dot. I do, however, know that he's one of the finest cyclists to come out of New Zealand and was one of the biggest transfers of the off-season at the end of 2021, moving from Primož Roglič's Jumbo–Visma to fierce rivals UAE Team Emirates.

The Kiwi spent seven seasons with the Dutch team before swapping canary yellow for the red, white and black livery of UAE Team Emirates. Bennett won the 2017 Tour of California but is now regarded as a super-domestique (the ultimate hod-carrier) and was one of eight riders brought in by the Emirates outfit alongside the likes of Movistar's Marc Soler and Quick-Step's João Almeida. Their strength in-depth is staggering. As is their budget – a reported €35 million in 2021. Only Ineos Grenadiers, at an annual €50 million, have such deep rear pockets.

Shortly before I interviewed Bennett at the start of January, I'd spent the Christmas period on the Isle of Wight. The occasional run and Boxing Day swim acted as informal training for L'Étape du Tour before I'd seek a structured, cycling-specific plan to follow from January to July. It offered brief respite from The Spyglass Inn, one of my favourite pubs, which sits at the western end of Ventnor Esplanade. The views of the English Channel are immense, as are the choice of real ales, nightly live music and seafood curry. It's conducive to fun, not fitness, and I returned to the mainland with a few more fatty deposits rolling over my belt. I wondered if Bennett, whose racing weight hovers around 58kg – or the weight of nine-year-old me – piled on similar festive surplus.

'Not necessarily at Christmas but my weight can fluctuate massively and when I jumped back on my bike after around a month off from early October, I was 5kg heavier,' he says. 'Much of that was down to drinking beer and bad food. My muscles ached a lot, too, from playing cricket and football. The key is to strip it down slowly; you don't want to crash diet and put yourself in a hole. That's where a lot of guys make mistakes – they don't eat enough.'

Not this writer.

Still, it's refreshing that elite cyclists aren't always the (extremely skinny) robots they're often portrayed as. Whether I can jettison the excess like Bennett remains to be seen, of course, especially as Bennett has the team's nutritionist, Gorka Prieto-Bellver, to call upon. 'He helps match the food and recipes to the training demands,' Bennett explains. 'And those demands have changed since I've moved teams. It turns out there are many ways to skin a cat when it comes to being a good cyclist. Jumbo had a blanket approach to training, really. It worked for Primož, it worked for Wout [van Aert], so they applied it to all.

'Here, UAE's really looked into the numbers, of the individualisation of training, and they noted that once I'd burnt through a certain amount of kilojoules, my performance dropped off. They really looked under the hood and, at the moment, I'm doing far fewer hours on the bike but much harder efforts. This time last year I was riding 30-hour weeks; last week I did 17 hours.' You remember I mentioned the ideal versus reality? I will in no way be cycling 30 hours a week. Or 17 hours. Maybe 10 max. Down the line. When I'm a shrinking, swifter version of myself. Again, hopefully, we will see...

Bennett's overhaul included strength work. In the past, he concedes that despite a growing body of evidence suggesting gym sessions should be an integral part of a cyclist's programme to bulletproof the body from injury and bolster power output, squats and lunges remained off-limits. 'Now, I'm in there two or three times a week. In fact, earlier in the off-season I was in there every day. It's very much specific to performance, so I'm doing lots of leg presses; I'm trying to rip up my muscles and grow them...' He looks down at his limbs and chuckles. 'But they haven't changed much. I guess I'm not that way [bulky] inclined. Still, it's a balancing act as I'm looking to build muscle but also to strip fat that I gained in the off-season.'

Clearly, there were lessons here for me. Potentially train at higher intensity, for fewer hours, and incorporate strength work and time in the gym. Got it.

Bennett didn't actually make it to the training camp in Alicante, instead remaining at home in New Zealand, the southern-hemisphere sun perfect for off-season miles. He lives in Nelson, a city on the eastern shores of Tasman Bay. There's a good 30-minute climb nearby that's his bread-and-butter, though his European base of Andorra is a world away, with mountainous adventures around every corner. He'll head there when the worst of the winter's over. It'll be warmer, meaning he'll avoid the modern cyclist's – certainly the modern recreational cyclist's – best friend: the indoor trainer. 'I used it during lockdown but after that I was ready to throw the damn thing out the window and never look at it again,' Bennett protests. 'I just find it dull.'

Bennett is seemingly in the minority. Lockdown made indoor trainers rarer than hen's teeth and saw online virtual software Zwift double its user base to over three million. Despite restrictions being lifted, it remains popular. I can see the merits of indoor cycling through the winter, so it's on my training radar. It's not now on Bennett's. The only time he spends indoor cycling is on an ergometer for fitness testing. He'd recently undertaken an hour test in a sports science laboratory in Girona, where he recorded an incredible VO_2 max score in the '90s. The average for someone of Bennett's age is about half that. VO_2 max is a measure of an individual's maximum lung capacity, reflecting their cardiovascular fitness, and is measured in millilitres of oxygen used by a kilogram of bodyweight every minute.

'It's an overrated gauge of performance, I feel,' says Bennett. 'No matter what your VO_2 is, it's how you arrive at the last climb. It's all about repeatability and efficiency. And it's about finding key positions and still being in good shape. Racing has changed. It's harder. Nowadays, riders are attacking with 60km to go and everyone's on their knees at the finish. Before, you'd let the break go, control things and race the last 5km. Of course, that still happens but there's been a definite shift from big hours to high-power stuff.'

And with that, Bennett looks at the time, interrupts himself and waves goodbye as he has to chow down on an energy bar and head out for a three-hour ride on his Colnago. Perhaps I should follow his example and dust off my saddle... There's little respite for the pros even with the Tour a mere hillock on the horizon, but Bennett's brief physiological overview whetted my appetite to know more about what it takes to race at the upper echelons. We sit on our sofas and watch as Ned Boulting and his team guide us vicariously around France in July but if you're anything like me, you'll want to know what has gone on behind the scenes. How many racing and training miles have the riders ticked off to make the team? How many calories have they burned through? How much chamois cream have they layered on? I need to answer these questions because, albeit in my own small way, I need to be ready for my own mini Tour de France.

Somebody who is well placed to answer some of these questions is Dr Daniel Green, performance consultant at Chris Froome's team, Israel–Premier Tech. Dr Green is a cycling whack-a-mole, popping up at one outfit before disappearing and popping up at another. As a cycling journalist, I've come across Green at the now disbanded BMC Racing and Team Qhubeka, Trek–Segafredo and now Israel. Every time I've spoken to him, I've understood why the modern cycling outfits battle for his services. He consumes data for breakfast and is a man who thrives on pacing strategies, aerodynamics and training loads. He's worked with the world's best and knows what it takes to elicit world-class performance.

During his time at BMC Racing, for example, Green undertook a project to understand exactly what it takes to make, survive and hopefully thrive in the WorldTour. 'At that time [2016–2018] we used SRM Power Meters,' Green explained when I interviewed him for this book. SRM is credited with creating the first cycling power meter – a device to measure power output of the rider – in 1986 to prescribe training sessions more accurately. Greg LeMond and Lance Armstrong became high-profile proponents and SRM continues to measure the world's finest. 'Taking data from there and using my own software, I analysed data files from all the riders from 1 November 2016 to September 2017. That was 327 days, comprising 8600 files and over 24,000 hours of data to pore over.

'What did I discover? Well, on average a WorldTour rider cycles for 876 hours a year. That equates to 27,500km, of which 326km is climbing. They expend 660,000kJ, broken down roughly as 14 per cent from anaerobic sources [hard], 49 per cent from aerobic sources [moderate] and 37 per cent from endurance load [easy]. Racing accounted for around 43 per cent of total load with training at 57 per cent. Of those 67 days' racing, intensity is generally higher than in training. Illness and injury came in at an average 14 days across the team.'

And so Green continued. But he needn't have. I got the hint. A snapshot was enough to offer a glimpse of how these bellows on saddles can cycle over 3200km around France every July, taming the biggest mountains of the Pyrenees and Alps, and still have enough energy to sprint down the Champs-Élysées on the final day of 21.

'The Tour wasn't actually the hardest race that year,' Green went on. 'That was the Vuelta a España. That adds up with the anecdotal [evidence] as the riders fed back that the heat made it particularly brutal. Relatively, the Giro d'Italia had the lowest workload of the three Grand Tours.'

'What about one-day races?' I asked, knowing that my own journey might feature a spring sportive in northern Europe. My challenge isn't solely about the end point (i.e. L'Étape du Tour) – in my watered-down way, I'm looking to mimic the professional calendar with two or three build-up events. 'A few stood out, notably Amstel Gold and Liège–Bastogne–Liège. They were the two biggest races of the year from a load point of view, which is surprising when you think of races like Paris–Roubaix and Tour of Flanders.'

(Mental note: do not sign up for sportives at either Amstel or Liège.)

The rise of the power meter provides fertile territory for the likes of Green to dig deep into the physiology of these superhumans. Or try to. The problem is that those 27,500km planted on a perch leave very little time for anything else, so the last thing most professional cyclists want to do is head over to a university and become a lab rat in their spare time.

Doing exactly that was clearly rather more in vogue in the 1990s, thanks to the infamous exploits of renowned drug cheats Dr Michele Ferrari, Festina, Armstrong and others involved in the infamous doping scandals of the time. As an aside, in researching this book I came across website 53x12.com, run by Dr Ferrari. In it, the disgraced Italian doctor provides tips on everything from supplements to enhance diet – 'Linseed oil is an alternative to fish oils' – to recovery – 'Try to do relaxing activities before you go to bed, such as taking a hot shower or listening to soothing music.' I couldn't find anywhere nefarious advice on injecting testosterone for muscle repair, and how best to avoid clotting from blood bags by awakening in the middle of the night to increase heart rate with a gentle walk around the hotel's corridors. As recently as 2019, he was linked to professional cyclists, with an undercover investigation by Cycling Anti-Doping Foundation (CADF) linking Ferrari and Astana's Alexey Lutsenko. Active riders found consulting with Ferrari could mean that they would face up to two-year bans, according to anti-doping rules.

But I digress. Professional cyclists' unsurprising reluctance to spend limited free time having muscle fibres extracted from their thighs means university students are the usual subjects used in sports science experiments all around the world. It's why a paper released in 2022, 'How do world-class top-five Giro d'Italia finishers train'[1], attracted so much attention in elite cycling circles. This kind of data is rare.

The team, led by Luca Filipas of the University of Milan, ostensibly followed a similar analytical template to Green's, unlocking the secrets of huge swathes of data emanating from power meters. The numbers were collected between 2015 and 2018, during which period each rider enjoyed at least one top-five Giro finish. It's a physiologist's nirvana, with standouts including: the riders' VO_2 max scores were 81, 82 and 80ml/min/kg, respectively; maximum 20-minute power output came in at 6.6, 6.6 and 6.4 watts per kg; and, surprisingly perhaps, training came in at 'just' 19.7, 16.2 and 14.7 hours on the bike each week, albeit much of this was during the race-preparation period when volume is generally lower. The paper also echoed Green's conclusions that the majority of training was low to medium intensity but when intensity was high, it was high. In other words, temple-pulsating, lung-squeezing high.

As were those VO_2 max scores. In Bennett's world, VO_2 max is no limiter because it's taken as read that to have reached WorldTour level, you're an oxygen-burning machine. For the rest of us, it's a clear proxy of fitness, a fitness badge of honour, or dishonour, depending on your score. You're probably wondering what my own VO_2 max score is? Hold fire on that one. My train of thought was still focused on the elite nirvana. More specifically, how high can VO_2 max reach before a ceiling's arrived at? I know there's a genetic ceiling but what's the highest that ceiling has ever reached?

It didn't take long – one Google search – to discover that Norwegian cyclist Oskar Svendsen recorded the highest-ever recorded VO_2 max score of 96.7ml/min/kg in 2012. Svendsen was only 18 years old at the time and this was more than double the average score of other male cyclists his age.

Impressive. But clearly no guarantee of success and fame as who the hell is Oskar Svendsen? Bennett's not-the-be-all-and-end-all of endurance performance maxim had substance: a search on ProCyclingStats – the stats site for cycling aficionados all around the world – revealed that Svendsen's last race was the Tour de l'Avenir in 2014, where he finished 71st overall. The Tour de l'Avenir is a micro-Tour de France for riders aged under 23 and is where agents and managers from around the globe gather to identify future stars. Past winners include Grand Tour winners Egan Bernal, Nairo Quintana, Miguel Induráin, Greg LeMond and Felice Gimondi. Svendsen, not looking overly happy in his bio pic, the name Joker stamped across his chest – he raced for Team Joker in Norway, which folded in 2020 due to financial pressures of Covid – never raced again, retiring at the tender age of 20.

So, just two years after that record-breaking VO_2 max score, his cycling career was done. Finito. No more. I couldn't let it lie. Why had someone with such potential, a machine whose lungs and heart are closer to those of a horse than a human, reached that performance ceiling so soon? I needed to know more, and soon found it via LinkedIn.

I messaged, we connected and Svendsen agreed to tell his story. 'Throughout that year, I'd undertaken several laboratory tests. Each time my VO_2 max scores were increasing. The first one was around 72, then 78, 80, 82, 87 and then 92...' Tour winners Bernal and Pogačar reportedly have scores around 89ml/kg/min. 'I then hit the labs in Lillehammer and undertook another test, reaching 96.7ml/kg/min...' That beat the world record set by cross-country star Bjorn Daehlie in the 1990s. 'It was a very strange atmosphere. The team around me had been screaming, but then it went quiet. I was thinking, "OK, what's happening now?" There was this awkward silence. They were then like, "Shit, there must be something wrong with the equipment". That's why they had it checked over by the distributors the following day, but it was calibrated correctly – the scores were correct.'

In physiological terms, Svendsen had broken cycling's hour record. Three weeks later, he won the men's junior time trial at the UCI Road World Championships, beating Slovenia's Matej Mohorič into second. Germany's Maximilian Schachmann took bronze.

Svendsen became hot property, appearing on Norwegian talk shows and becoming a regular on the radio. He was talked about as the new Thor Hushovd, who won the Worlds in 2010. But while Mohorič and Schachmann would both go on to secure lucrative WorldTour contracts, Svendsen would return to his studies before taking up a role at a Norwegian start-up that makes automated systems for herbs and vegetables.

'It was a crazy time. I'd only been cycling for three years [Svendsen was an alpine skier before then] and things felt out of my control. A lot of professional teams were watching me and I ended up signing for Continental side Team Joker. But I had a real comedown and lost motivation.' The media spotlight frazzled and the idea of further adulation was blinding. He chose to end his career before it had really begun.

Svendsen still rides for leisure and can revel in the fact that he's the fittest grocer who's ever lived (albeit Gregg Wallace might contest otherwise, as the TV presenter now has a six-pack and runs a fitness site called Showme.fit, on which Gregg offers his pearls of wisdom for £7 a month).

So, fitness matters, but you're an empty shell if the elite mindset is cracked or you simply don't like or want the attention. This is where your environment matters. It needs to be conducive to world-class performance but not so stressful that you can't escape the world's gaze. Which brings us back to Alicante, off-season road-cycling training, and my mission.

Until the 2020 pandemic, the Costa Blanca had become an annual pilgrimage, a place where I researched, conducted interviews and wrote features about cycling for various publications especially *Cyclist* magazine. I recall strolling around a hotel on the edge of Calpe in search of Belgian team Quick-Step's press officer Alessandro Tegner. Alessandro is all tan, slicked-back black hair and unflappable confidence. There are no specifics with Alessandro but, he assured me, the day I'd requested to observe the world's most successful cycling team was sorted. 'It's always sorted,' he'd deliver with easy charm. Sadly, we had form. Bad form. Of photo shoots and interviews lined up, only for our media arrival to coincide with said rider departure. 'Next time,' Alessandro would repeat casually. 'It'll all be good next time.' The editor, staring at eight blank pages and the imminent iceberg that is a print deadline, lacked Alessandro's leisurely spirit.

To be fair to Alessandro, managing the media commitments of naturally introverted riders as they compete all over the world is no easy task. Thankfully, their sometime ambivalence towards the press is matched by a laser focus that ignores the tacky temptations abundant in this part of Spain. Calpe and Dénia are next to Benidorm and are its pubescent siblings. Calpe, in particular, is all late-night dentist chairs and beer-bellied Brits, albeit without the omnipresence of high-rise hotels that scar its elder brother. 'This area is an example of man gone bad,' lamented photographer Juan Trujillo Andrades when I'd first visited this off-season cycling playground. 'The Costa Blanca is such a beautiful part of Spain. Well, it was. Then Benidorm happened.'

Benidorm was the original Dubai. In the 1950s, the entire town had just 102 hotel rooms. That was before Mayor Pedro Zaragoza Orts set about transforming Benidorm into Europe's first tourist hotspot, writing into law a series of rules and regulations designed to attract sun-seeking northern Europeans. He turned a blind eye to religious objections and even convinced Franco that opening Benidorm's door to tourism would provide welcome pesetas for the entire country. According to the *Economist* magazine's[2] obituary of Orts in April 2008, 'The dictator, amused by this small, round moustachioed man with motor oil on his trousers, became a fan.' Franco signed off on the developments, and even encouraged the high-rises so more people could see the beaches and breathe in the sea air.

Calpe and Dénia followed a similar, though less aggressive, path, making them an incongruous backdrop to the planet's fittest and most svelte human beings, for whom sub-10 per cent body fat is the norm. They head to these parts for winter's traffic-free roads, stiff climbs and affordable hotels. Which is a rather odd juxtaposition within the respective hotel's dining area, where all that separates the power-packed, tanned cyclists and red-faced tourists is a wafer-thin partition.

I recall from pre-Covid visits how on one side you had retired Brits tucking into two words that arouse even the most committed narcoleptic: 'buffet breakfast'. Knowing their market, the continental had been dropped; there was no slither of ham, triangular cheese, bread roll and rock-solid pot of butter here. When in Rome – or Calpe – eat English. And what a feast. Anaemic bacon sought CPR in the oil of overcooked eggs, nestled against crinkled sausages and, a conciliatory nod to health, the heavily baked tomato that steadfastly refused to cool down. Consume, go up for more, consume. And there were no worries if your appetite is not satiated – this is all-inclusive calories 24/7. On the other side of the partition sat riders tucking into porridge, nuts, rice and fruit. Healthy, performance-based, fast.

On which side should I sit? Back then, I'd be wrestling with the buffet. If Covid had allowed me to attend now, that tendency to gluttony and my erratic training would have to change if I was to reach my goal of completing the Étape. Despite Bennett's protestations, VO_2 max *is* important. It's a gauge of how quickly your lungs, heart and muscles can process oxygen. So, the lighter you are, the higher you'll score. It was time to assess where I was and, once the tears of disappointment had dried, I would need a plan. That assessment, I felt, was going to be an eye-opener and rather painful...

'This sat-nav's playing with me. It's playing with me, I tell you!' Destination Liverpool John Moores University, for a series of physiological tests. It's named after Sir John Moores, a local businessman and philanthropist. In short, it's a mainstay, established ... and it's currently disappeared from the map. The network of roads into the city has confused the technology – it won't be the last time on this Étape journey – and bookends a typically chaotic morning.

It's mid-January. It's raining. I woke late, had to put out the bins and, in the rush to head north from my Bristol home, I think I've forgotten my bike shoes. I'd received a fleeting motivational boost from interviewing Bennett and Green, which had been swiftly snuffed out by life, the universe and everything. Work's manic, family are, well, family, and the remnants of my festive weight gain cling on for dear life. I mentally and physically feel like Mr Blobby. All I need now for this day to be complete is for Noel Edmonds (whom I once met at the Bitton beer festival) to chase me around Liverpool, slapping my derrière with that cheeky grin of his.

I was here to be measured. And I wouldn't be able to avoid the results. 'Relax before the day's events to maximise the results' the physiological brief read. Chance would be a fine thing.

Thankfully, my sat-nav and I recalibrate. I arrive at the Tom Reilly Building, which is the sports science arm of Liverpool John Moores. I remember reading about Tom Reilly in my academic days, when I was one of a handful of folk to study English Literature and Sport Science at the University of Worcester.

Professor Tom Reilly undertook the first thesis on the physiology of football back in the 1970s. His PhD involved analysing the match demands of Everton Football Club but this was long before a GPS-inserted vest could track every player's sprint, jog or stepover; instead, diligent Tom would be in the stands and hand-note distances covered by the players and the percentages of the game they spent running with the ball. I know this detail thanks to the man who welcomed me into the Tom Reilly Building, Mr James Morton.

Morton is professor of exercise metabolism, and a busy man. On top of authoring more than 160 research publications, he was the performance nutritionist for Liverpool FC between 2010 and 2015. After that, he headed up nutrition and physical performance support at Team Sky, playing a pivotal role in the British team's four successive Tour de France victories between 2015 and 2018.

I've come across Morton numerous times over the years, including at a Team Sky Mallorcan training camp, where he went into great detail about how to maximise fasted training. It's something I'll look to apply to my own performance, but more on that later. He's a charismatic figure, Morton, his chiselled cheeks, shaved head and piercing eyes complementing his soft Irish brogue. He has something of the Bond villain about him…

'Hello James, we've been expecting you.' A mind-reader, too.

As a favour to help me research this book, he has booked me in for a day of fitness testing to gauge just how far I'll have to climb to reach my goals. I am no Chris Froome. I need to lose a few pounds. I am, however, fuelled by distorted sporting memories; of times when, if the stars had aligned – and I hadn't accidentally headbutted my fellow central defender – I could have been a professional footballer. It was a south-west football trial for Watford. I tell people this story. Half my team had a trial for Watford. I don't tell them this. It dilutes the achievement. Once, in my head, I was closer to the elite sportsmen whom I now report on. That's how I remember it. Like I said, time could easily have distorted those memories. Either way, today's the day of truth.

'The day will have four components to it,' explains Morton. 'We'll start by looking at your body composition and then move on to resting metabolic rate. They're the easy ones as they require no effort. The next two do – as we'll examine your aerobic physiology and maximal physiology. All of this impacts your cycling performance.

'Right, let's look at your body composition via a set of scales and bioelectrical impedance. So, if you'd like to pop your clothes on the side, that'd be grand.'

I beg your pardon? Clearly, I hadn't read the small print. But I'm wearing the oldest, tiredest pair of boxer shorts I own; I suspect my mum bought them from the local market 25 years ago. Some might see this as lacking self-respect; I see it as being ahead of the planet-saving game, though I don't want to advertise the fact in public. Still, there'll be plenty of humbling hurdles to drag myself over during the next six months. I might as well start with the most undignified.

I mount the scales, grab the handles and data flashes up in front of me. The device is similar to what you might find in a leisure centre but more accurate, more reliable and more expensive. 'OK, those results are … OK,' says Morton. Hmmm, I'm no psychologist but I'm sure when the likes of Olympic gold medallist triathlete Alistair Brownlee tested here, they didn't receive an 'OK'.

'Right, you weigh 91kg, of which total body fat is around 20kg.' So, I've lost a kilogram since the weigh-in since I signed up for L'Étape the previous month but it still makes me suspiciously closer to a pork scratching than a human being. 'It's fine,' says Morton. Hmm… Height is 188m (which is odd as I thought I was 1.89m. I'm shrinking). 'Results can be affected by hydration and you're coming up dehydrated.'

Thirsty? I'm parched. As well as encouraging this mythical pre-test rest, I'm sure it had said to refrain from drinking for several hours beforehand. I'm a big water drinker – in turn, a big urinator – and was increasingly aware of my breathing. I see breathing like a good football referee – if it's doing its job proficiently, you shouldn't even notice it.

This awareness grew in part two, which required me to lie down (my clothes were back on by now) on a medical-looking bed and have a dome placed over my sizeable head (I once had a helmet mapped to my dimensions and my cranium was in the top 5 per cent, #proud), with a stretch of material that resembled a transparent poncho draped over my upper body. A tube around 10cm in diameter was connected to the dome, from which my metabolic rate would be analysed.

'It's called an indirect calorimeter and will require you to chill for around 20 minutes. It works by assessing the amount of heat generated according to the amount of substrates used and by-products generated.' The results will provide a base figure you can use when you're looking to hit race weight. I was then left to it and, for the first time that day, I relaxed. And drifted. It was similar to a flotation tank I'd once visited with my wife, where salt and water had eased the pressure from gravity while darkness further nullified the senses. It had been incredibly cleansing until some of the salt had seeped into my eyes.

Back on the bed, I sensed the door opening. 'OK, we're done.' Damn – I could have stayed in there all day, especially as I knew the sedentary part of the assessment was over. 'Your metabolic rate at rest, which means how many calories you burn to perform everyday functions like breathing, is 1824kcal.' So, I can eat one extremely large roast every day and not put on an ounce. I might as well go home...

On to the next test. 'All good?' Morton asks me. 'Moderate,' is my response, muffled by the gas-analysis mask that had been strapped to my face for the past 15 minutes while I undertook a fitness test. I was lying. The actual riding itself was OK. It was the thick plastic muzzle that was causing the problems, disrupting my breathing rate and nudging anxiety. This was clearly a test for fetishists.

This masochism was all in the name of understanding my physical capabilities. We decided on just doing a sub-maximal test instead of full-on maximal test. I can't begin to tell you how happy this made me. Even the professionals dislike the maximal fitness test. Coach Dan Healey, formerly of WorldTour team Tinkoff–Saxo, who are now no more but shone bright for a while thanks to their outrageous billionaire owner Oleg Tinkov, told me that he doesn't even bother with them now. 'If I mention it to riders, individuals who are being paid millions of pounds per year, they look at you and say, "Do I really fucking need to do this test? No? Good."' It takes you to the limits and is messy. Very messy.

This is no irrational fear. At school, I like many before me and many after regularly undertook the beep test. I see you shudder, for the beep test, or 'multi-stage fitness test' to give it its mildly more formal moniker, was designed to satiate the sadistic appetite of aged and nefarious PE teachers to humiliate adolescent schoolchildren.

That's how I saw it anyway as my brethren and I would reluctantly change into ill-fitting, cost-effective, mud-stained cotton sports attire, tramp over to the frozen, drenched fields of Devon in December, and run up and down at ever-increasing speeds. Over a distance of

20m, you'd jog from one end to the other to arrive before the beep. Over time, the gap between the beeps would close in, like that wall in *Indiana Jones*. So would the gaps between each breath. You ran and then sprinted until you could either no longer keep up with the beeps or you'd avoided the ignominy of quitting first. You'd then quit, blaming your recently diagnosed but hitherto never-revealed asthma. (By my reckoning, 95 per cent of the students who went to my school between 1989 and 1993 said they had asthma. The field was a wheezing sea of blue-and-brown inhaler lids. I suspect doctors were on commission from big pharma.)

I've never formed a beep-test self-help group, never sought beep-test therapy, so I don't recall my scores. I do recall that Carl Hagerty, lovely chap, always finished top. At a professional level, Seb Coe was reported as top beeper at 17. As was a Kiwi rugby player whose name escapes me.

Back to the present day. I was in the much less exposing environment of the labs and, on a cycle ergometer, faced a screen featuring variables including heart rate, cadence (how many times you pedal each minute), pedal efficiency and power output (in watts). As for that suffocating mask, it was there to measure fuel utilisation. This determines the split of fat and carbohydrate fuelling a rider's efforts at different intensities. If you can ride hard and predominantly burn fat, you're in a good place, as even the pros have tonnes of the stuff. Carbohydrate, on the other hand, is stored as glycogen, of which you have a maximum 2000kcal stored in your muscles, liver and brain.

I started on an easy 100 watts, which increased by 20 watts every four minutes, at the end of which increment blood was taken from the end of my finger to assess lactate content (a sign of how hard I'm working and something we'll look into further in Chapter 4). Morton also recorded my heart rate while I shouted out how I was feeling. This was to measure my rate of perceived exertion and scaled from an easy 1 to a balls-out 10. Being a sub-maximal test, this didn't edge over 7 but, as the stream of sweat revealed, it was still taxing.

'You'll see some VO_2 max numbers on there, too, but these represent a predicted value, extrapolated from the sub-max response, so take this with a pinch of salt. More important is the fractional utilisation. In other words, the first lactate threshold [the maximum level of exercise intensity or blood lactate that the body can withstand for a period of time]. What I say to a customer is you have your VO_2 max. That is the upper limit of your performance. But arguably, it's more vital what percentage of that VO_2 max you can sustain before it all falls apart.' This links to Bennett's assertions that having the ability to go hard and go again is a better indicator of performance than aerobic capacity. But, clearly, I'd like both.

The first lactate treshold, or aerobic threshold – although the exact definition is somewhat debated – relates to the average power that can be maintained for around three hours. After brief analysis, mine came in at 160 watts. The report also signalled moderate fat-burning potential and an over-reliance on carbohydrates at a relatively low intensity. Not great. 'Longer sessions will help shift this balance and there's glycogen-depleted efforts [training without being fuelled], though keep these to a minimum.'

'So, are we done?' I ask. 'Maybe,' Morton replies. 'But we do have time for the maximal test if you're interested?' Morton, you sadist. Hmm, I'm no type-A but I am competitive enough that the thought of not digging deeper and discovering my VO_2 max was a dangling carrot that I was ready to munch on. Once I'd removed the mask for a breather, of course.

'This time, we'll start from around where you finished the last test. That's around 245 watts. Every minute, I'll increase that by 25 watts. We don't need to collect blood this time but you will need that mask back on. The test is terminated when your cadence drops below 70rpm. Are you ready?'

I'm sure that's what Marie-Antoinette was asked at the Place de la Révolution. And with that, and with the asphyxiator back in place, I was away. Mentally, physically and emotionally. The first minute passed without incident, the second began to chafe ... and after that it was just a hazy fog. I was a sweaty lump and my lungs, then mouth, were making some rather distressing whistling noises. Every minute, that Rated Perceived Exertion (RPE) scale ramped up until the guillotine dropped and my mind, body and soul left the building.

'Good effort,' Morton says. True or not, as I was shellshocked, positive affirmation right then was jolly appreciated. 'You terminated at around 375 watts, leaving your VO_2 max at 47. That's pretty good.'

'Pretty good?' Morton was clearly now my new best friend. In fact, a scan online and a chart informed me that my score was 'good'. Let's drop the 'pretty'. It was not excellent – for a 45-year-old, excellent is around 50 and clearly not up there with Oskar, George and co. But this trip up north had nevertheless been a worthwhile exercise, if not a roller-coaster one, starting with my exposure on the scales and finishing with a gentle stroke of the ego. George might not think the VO_2 max is that important, but what does a professional cyclist with 10 years' experience racing at the top level, racking up hundreds of thousands of cycling kilometres over the world's biggest mountain ranges, know?

I'd need to spend time unpicking these terms, the figures and the repercussions but it was immediately clear that I needed to cut weight. I was easily over 89kg and felt every kilo during both tests. Oxygen simply couldn't reach the parts I needed it to. There was too much to fuel and not enough of an engine to fuel it. Still, keep chipper, I told myself. I needed the open mindset that's the cornerstone of everyone with ambition and going places. If I hadn't measured it, how could I improve it? This was the new me, one of whom renowned psychologist and mindset expert Carol Dweck would be proud. I'll summon my inner Dan Walker, my inner Jake Humphreys, for whom disappointment hits a wall against their positive attitude and perma-smiles. There'll be no Scotch egg on the drive home. Now, it's all about malt loaf, water and, of course, riding a bike. But before then, I needed a plan. I got out my contacts list and emailed Phil Mosley, coach and training expert.

'Phil, you're a man and I need a plan. Can you help?' Of course Phil can help. He is one of the nicest humans I've come across. I remember covering Phil's exploits when I reported on triathlon. He then took up the coaching mantle and has spent the past 20 years or so training recreational cyclists, triathletes and runners to reach their goals without ending up in the divorce court. 'My plans ensure you'll have quality time available for family, friends and career,' Phil's bio reads. 'As a parent who works for a living, I know how challenging this can be.'

That's key to this whole no-pro project. I've interviewed countless amateur endurance athletes over the years who seemingly think nothing of training for upwards of 20 hours a week. They'll cruise down the finish line and lift their young children up in the air in celebration. The youngsters are beaming, but the cynic in me suspects this familial joy is more down to the kids seeing their mother or father for the first time in months rather than awestruck delight at their achievement. Maybe I'm wrong. Maybe I'm just envious of their ability to juggle. Either way, I'm after a plan that'll lead to peak progress but not at the expense of relationship distress.

'I have just the plan for you,' Phil said. 'It's a 100-miler and aimed at beginners.' How rude. 'Don't be offended – I know you've done endurance events before but it'll suit what you're after. It's 24 weeks long and even at its peak will consume no more than 10 hours a week.'

Perfect. 'Is there anything you'd like to ask before I detail the plan?' Yes, Phil, there is. Every Monday night for years, Goals five-a-side complex at Brislington in Bristol has echoed to the grunts and gasps of myself and nine other chaps of my age reliving our youths. It's around 75 minutes of high-octane, debatable-skill activity that I ruddy love. Football was my first passion and continues to loom large in my life. I love meeting my mates, the competition, the exercise without thinking you're exercising and the pure reward for getting through a Monday.

I don't enjoy the fact that the adrenaline from middle-aged competition and occasional sprinting kills sleep of a Monday eve and takes me around three days to recover from. It's totally worth the physical and mental degradation but is it conducive to a consistent training plan? Please say it is, Phil.

'It'll only become a problem if you get injured.' Fair point, and one that reminds me of football-related broken ankle, wrist and ribs.

But still, one-offs… 'With the plan, you won't be riding every day, so it's manageable. You might have to move sessions around as you wouldn't want to follow an intense football match on the Monday with an intense bike on the Tuesday as you'll be too fatigued and could end up side-lined. The whole point of this plan is that it fits in around your life, not totally absorbs it.'

Praise be, Phil. And actually, what was I worried about? An increasing number of WorldTour riders have even integrated running into their training programmes. OK, football's a different beast to jogging but it'll still deliver the physiological benefits that the likes of Primož Roglič, Mike Woods and Tom Pidcock are after.

Roglič's coach, Mathieu Heijboer, who used to train George Bennett, once told me that every day without fail, even during the race season, Roglič will start the day with a 20–30-minute run. 'It's something he carried over from his ski-jumping days and he feels better for an early morning run,' the Dutchman said.

You can see why. While cycling elicits myriad health benefits, bone density isn't one of them; in fact, Chris Boardman retired at just 32 years of age due to cycling-fuelled osteoporosis. Studies show that weight-bearing and impact exercise like running is what researchers term an 'effective osteogenic stimulus', which leads to improved bone health. Cycling is a non-weight-bearing activity, meaning there's no stimulus, raising the spectre of debilitating conditions like osteoporosis. A 2011 study[3] by Doctor Kyle Nagle showed that cyclists have particularly poor health in the neck and lumbar spine. But not Roglič. 'For a GC rider, he has remarkable bone density,' Heijboer continued. 'In fact, he's rarely injured – not overuse injuries anyway – which again goes back to his ski-jump training where he'd do a lot of co-ordination and balance work.'

If it's good enough for them…

So, what of the plan beyond Monday ball-bashing? As a reminder, my goal is L'Étape du Tour on 10 July. It's just under 170km long and features 4700m of climbing. With that in mind, back to Phil… 'There are two goals to the plan. The first is that by the end of the plan you'll be able to ride for over five hours without feeling like you need to spend the rest of the day in bed. That means one long ride each week. At first, you might ride for a couple of hours and feel knackered. But you'll become used to it as you grow stronger.

'The other goal is to build up your FTP or functional threshold power. We'll test this every eight weeks. The higher your FTP, the faster you'll be able to ride five hours without spending all day in bed. To achieve this, we'll have a mix of threshold and sub-threshold sessions during the week but they're rarely longer than an hour, hour and a half. In short, building endurance and your FTP are the main goals.'

From a recent test on my mate's smart trainer (an interactive turbo trainer that feeds data to an app), I knew my FTP was around 215 watts (I hadn't covered this in my Liverpool tests because it would all have been too much on one day). I'd also spent a few weeks riding to and from Bristol to Clevedon (about 65km) in preparation for what Phil informed me was the preparation phase. This would last four weeks and was designed to acclimatise me to following a training programme. 'For some people, finding a routine and making it work within the rest of their lives is a shock to the system. The key is that you find the right places and right times to train. The preparation phase is about sorting your equipment, about setting up bike computers. It won't be super hard, though it will involve four or five sessions a week. But if you miss a session, it's really not the end of the world. But before you do anything, I'd really recommend seeking out a professional for a bike fit and trying to sort a power meter as the plan is on power-meter software TrainingPeaks.'

OK, sort a bike fit. And preferably an affordable one, as they're not cheap. After the preparation phase, we'd crank things up but, as Phil said, never beyond 10 hours a week with shorter sessions in the week. (For more on the specifics of my training, *see* Appendix 1 from p. 252.)

2

Stolen Dreams

T-minus six months

'Remco Evenepoel. The emotion breaks over him. Liège crowns the wonderkid of Belgium as he takes his first Monument…' Broadcaster FloBikes' commentator couldn't contain his excitement as Remco Evenepoel, touted as the next in a long line of replica Eddy Merckx, won April 2022's Liège–Bastogne–Liège. The oldest cycling classic in the world, founded in 1892 just four years after John Boyd Dunlop invented the pneumatic tyre, had a new star. A beaming Evenepoel, peak of cap raised to display the sponsor logos of Quick-Step Floors and Alpha Vinyl, appraised his effort thus: 'I woke up with a really great feeling … until attacking over Côte de La Redoute, I hadn't felt my legs. I felt fresh.' The foundations for his 29km solo masterclass lay in limbs and torso conserving energy, of reducing drag and maximising power output for the least effort.

Rewind five months to November 2021 and Evenepoel is planted in front of an oversized turbine within the confines of bike manufacturer Specialized's Californian wind-tunnel to examine his road position in search of free speed and injury reduction. It's the latest off-season, high-tech step in the Specialized performance plan – to bulletproof their riders' bodies in preparation for the near 30,000km of annual pedalling ahead.

Professional bike-fitting is big business, with the merest relaxation of the elbow or lifting of the forearm potentially the difference between victory and defeat. But where once the likes of Merckx and his mechanic tinkered by feel – to the extent of changing saddle height on the fly – now it's all about the cutting edge.

'On the WorldTour, we work with three teams – Quick-Step, Bora–Hansgrohe and Total Energies,' explains Jason Williams, Retül bike-fitter at the Specialized Experience Center in Boulder, Colorado. Retül is regarded as a leading technological light in the world of bike-fitting – so much so that Specialized, who turn over half a billion dollars annually, bought them out in 2012. I'd set up an interview with Williams with half an eye on the pros' performance and two eyes on mine.

'There are potentially three to five pit-stops during the winter where my team and I will work with the riders, utilising a range of top-end equipment so they're optimising their time on the bike,' adds Williams. 'And it all starts after the World Championships [in September].

'In October, the teams have generally concluded their business and confirmed rider line-up for the following season, so that'll be where we'll spend time with the new riders setting them up with all their new equipment. Beyond bikes, that also means shoes and helmets.'

This is bike porn for the recreational roadie as the likes of Quick-Step's 2022 new recruits Martin Svrček, Louis Vervaeke and Mauro Schmid were fitted for the Specialized Tarmac road bike. Each rider is given three of these bikes at the beginning of the season: one for home, one for training camps and one for races. They also get three Specialized Shiv time trial bikes, plus more shoes than Imelda Marcos as well as aero, road and aero road helmets. That's a lot of bikes to fit each season for Williams' team of bike-fitters.

It's marginal sporting gains mingling with corporate hospitality. 'We usually meet up in a hotel located near the team's service course [operational base], which in the case of Quick-Step is Wevelgem,' Williams explains. 'There, we'll take over a handful of meeting rooms or a wedding banquet hall that we'll clear and [where we'll] set up three fitting stations so we can work with riders simultaneously.'

I recall a winter training camp where I was reporting on the now-disbanded CCC Racing team in Dénia, Spain, where a subterranean closed casino served as the bike-fit backdrop. Roulette and Blackjack tables were shoved into dark corners to be replaced by sensors and 3D cameras. The cycling croupier that day was Lloyd Thomas, who remained poker-faced over American Will Barta's position before declaring 'Textbook fluiddddddity' as the recent graduate from Pro Continental level pleased his master. That had been three years earlier. Barta is still a professional, now racing for Movistar Team.

The October bike fit is open to existing riders, too, but the majority eye flights to sun-kissed sands for a brief post-season break. They need it as, into November, things crank up with the next step in the fitting evolution, albeit strictly invite only. 'That's when the team will decide which riders they'll want to come over to our wind-tunnel in Morgan Hill,' says Williams. 'These tend to be riders who have a major role in the squad, like GC contenders or uber-domestiques.'

At the end of 2021, the winds of progress blew over young Evenepoel, who justified the tunnel's running costs with that 2022 Liège victory, plus Kasper Asgreen and Mattia Cattaneo. Asgreen is one of the strongest and most reliable support riders in the peloton, who occasionally diverts the spotlight on to himself, as in April 2021 when he outsprinted Mathieu van der Poel to victory at the Tour of Flanders. Cattaneo has a similar profile to Asgreen.

'This is where we're looking for miniscule improvements on the road and in TT [time trials],' Williams explains. 'It's a really impressive set-up because smack bang next to the tunnel is the human performance lab where we'll physiologically test the load on the riders in their refined position. We measure them in the wind-tunnel before applying those bike dimensions to the Fit bike in the lab, where they'll have a mask fitted and hit a certain power output in that position. From there, we can analyse the metabolic cost of that position. We're aiming for a combination of physiological efficiency and good aero numbers. If a position's aero but not sustainable, it's not aero.'

For two months, a drip-feed of riders undergo positional assessment. Come December, there's a full wave as for the only time in the year every rider in the squad – a maximum of 31 in the men's WorldTour in 2022 (dropping to 30 in 2023) and 20 in the women's – plus the near-100 support staff of mechanics, soigneurs, chefs and trainers gather for their respective team's pre-Christmas training camp.

'With Quick-Step, this is usually in Calpe,' says Williams. 'We'll check in with the new riders and see how they've settled into any positional changes, ensuring gear like the shoes and saddle is working for them. The training workload's increasing then so there'll be greater stress on their position, so it's a good benchmark for how sustainable and strong that set-up is. We'll see the existing riders, too, though only around 50 per cent. Many of the more experienced riders, who've enjoyed success, are disinclined to make a change. Then again, there are older riders who are right tinkerers. Those riders, whether in the pro or amateur ranks, keep us in work because even if we don't do anything, they want a once-over. "Let's try two millimetres down, two millimetres up. Any change? No? No worries."'

George Bennett, who we came across earlier, put it another way with typically Antipodean eloquence. 'When I moved from Jumbo–Visma to UAE [Team Emirates], I changed bike from Cervelo to Colnago. I had new pedals, new helmet, new saddle, new shoes … and yes, everything feels different. For a week you think about adjusting this, that and the other but after a couple of weeks of fighting it, you settle in. I'm lucky as I know plenty of guys who are unbelievably neurotic about position. They'll even carry an Allen key in their pocket at a race. Crazy. The only thing I *had* to swap was a saddle for one that wouldn't give me saddle sores or a vasectomy!'

Ahh, saddle sores, two words that are the butt of many a joke, until you get them. Then, the laughing stops. Along with the pedalling. I once interviewed Sean Kelly for *Cyclist* magazine (issue 79, October 2018) for a piece celebrating 30 years of his Vuelta a España victory. 'I could have won it before but I had a big boil on my bottom,' he told me. 'I was leading and there was just one big mountain stage left, but

I'd been managing the pain for six days and it just grew too painful. The team talked about putting a beef steak in my bib shorts to ease things but I didn't try that one. I slathered on creams and hoped that it would ease but when you're riding your bike for five hours every day, coupled with the hot weather, it just doesn't heal. It was difficult to take.'

At another race I was covering a few years ago, cycling doctor Dag Van Elslande invited me into the team bus and greeted me with a range of tubs, tubes and dressings. 'This is tar. I'm going to put it up your ass.' Silence. 'I'm joking – here's some for your finger. It's for saddle sores. It ripens an abscess faster and includes cod liver oil, zinc, disinfectant, vitamin E… We also have a local anaesthetic; a healing cream with zinc; Compeed, which acts as a second skin; Betadine soap that prevents your groin from picking up an infection…' To the aroma of a recently tarmacked road, I exited the bus, innocence lost.

The camp isn't just about the Retül fitting, of course. Cycling teams extract every last fiscal ounce from their off-season camps, like a chef who'll respect the slain animal by cooking everything, including the giblets.

'At the end of the camp, we'll head over to Valencia with many of the riders for further positional testing,' says Williams. 'It's not an amazing velodrome – it's basically a concrete track – but it works for aero-testing purposes.'

We'll delve deeper into the lengths the professionals go to in search of slipstreaming savings in Chapter 6. Plus, of course, any I can cherry-pick to satiate my own aero appetite. But that communication point is important. As alluded to, the WorldTour en masse meet up incredibly infrequently and it's easy to see how many progressive ideas could simply not come to fruition. It's why Sir Dave Brailsford set up a delivery unit in 2017 with the help of Tony Blair's former advisor, Sir Michael Barber, to help the British team work through issues that arise from daily performance meetings. An example would be something as simple as rapidly remedying riders who might have a puncture.

This focus on improving communication for better delivery is why Trek–Segafredo became the first team to bring in a full-time sport psychologist in the 2021 off-season. It's not just about the mechanical when it comes to training camps – it's about the mental, too. 'Training camps are super busy,' explained Italian psychologist Elisabetta Borgia. 'In one week, we had 150 people to potentially work with.' I'd set up an interview with Borgia to both understand the growing awareness of the pros' anxieties and whether I could boost my mind to help my legs pedal quicker!

Borgia works with riders individually, though much of her work is around team building. That's why she'll also work with the directeurs sportifs (DSes) and coaches on effective communication – about how to speak to the riders or how to host an effective pre-race meeting.

'I'm also an organisational psychologist. So, my job is to create systems and connect. For example, at a training camp, before I see the riders I'll ask about the soigneurs and mechanics. How are they feeling? Good or bad? Give them value in order to be validated and seen. The riders are the stars but we are all a team. It's why communication is so important.'

Interestingly, the work of experts like Williams could inadvertently load further pressure on the riders. Professional riders have everything measured, from their position to core temperature to their power output. 'But so many variables can cause problems,' said Borgia. 'If you have one or two variables to work on, you can deal with them, it's fine. But 100 of them can seem insurmountable, demotivating and cause stress.'

This is compounded by social media, meaning riders have few 'off' moments. 'The risk of burnout is super heavy, super hard,' says Borgia. 'Many riders have come to me in the past and ask[ed] me how to deal with social media. I can't be focused on my performance as I look at the others and don't feel good when I see my competitor doing 200km on Strava or whatever. That 24/7 comparison wasn't there in the past.

'How many big riders have had mental issues in these last three or four years? Take Marcel Kittel, for instance. It's important with the younger riders to help them to be aware of their emotions. Maybe they can perform as professional riders but many are teenagers and need to grow as people, not just riders. How many young riders have panic attacks? A lot. How many young riders have eating disorders? A lot. Why? Because they're not aware of their emotions, not aware of the origins of their emotions. It's an important part. Everyone only looks at the performance, at the bike, but it's more than that – you must create a positive culture.'

For some, that culture must be nurtured. For others, it's natural. 'I remember Mads Pederson at training camp went to McDonald's and bought 60 hamburgers for the staff after training. For him, it's all about the detail.'

And that detail matters, whether it's the explicit, like bike positioning and what Williams does, or the unseen work of the likes of Borgia. When it comes to a bike fit, I'd been convinced this too could benefit me, since Mosley insisted on me having one. Understanding the good work of Williams and co. made this desire greater. It was to be no refinement of a Ferrari, though. This would be an overhaul of the bike equivalent of a much-loved but much-used and abused Ford Cortina. But I hadn't thought of speaking to a sports psychologist. Our time is up for the interview, so I mentally set it aside as an area I might come back to. However, before Borgia returns to her clinic, where away from the sports arena she treats troubled youngsters, I ask for one snippet of advice for a rather tired, ageing 45-year-old no-pro.

'You mustn't copy the professional riders' training. Your energy tank is not unlimited. You have a job, other hobbies, maybe wake up early and have a full day. I see many recreational riders who would like to be professional and try and cram in the hours. Don't do that. Accept your situation. It might actually be better to do less than more…'

Thank you, Elisabetta. I will have 'do less than more' tattooed on to my forehead.

It's 5.30 a.m. and only the foxes and darkness accompany me as I ride to Bristol Temple Meads station to catch a train to Newport, and from there on to Manchester. It's an indirect route to avoid a severe hit to my bank account. Flirt with Wales and add an hour for £56; travel as the crow flies and it's more than double that figure. Inconvenience is fiscally convenient.

From Manchester Central, my bike and I will commute the 3.2km to the impressive Manchester Institute of Health and Performance, which was born from an Industrial Revolution hinterland that's been decontaminated and transformed by modern UAE money. I've been here before to uncover the sports-science secrets behind Pep Guardiola's game-changing style of tiki-taka football at Manchester City FC. It's a place of football pitches forged from artificial Desso grass, cryotherapy chambers and bespoke hydration strategies. While there previously, I'd noticed an altitude chamber that had cycling connections: Team Sky – I couldn't find out which rider – had booked a session to acclimate to the rarefied air of the upcoming Vuelta a España.

It transpires that the Institute is bristling with cycling innovation as well as football. Biomechanical, physiological, aerodynamic … it's all here to make you more efficient and that bit faster, a team of experts ready to mould you into a better version of you. And it's a former Team Sky stalwart who'll soon be manipulating my Devonian limbs with his burly Cornish paddles. Phil Burt was formerly the physio for Sir Bradley Wiggins, Geraint Thomas et al at both Team Sky and British Cycling. He was an original member of the Secret Squirrel Club, the team charged with technical development who took their name from a cartoon spy character.

Phil has had his hands on and sized up the world's greatest cyclists. Having had his fill of the nomadic lifestyle, he went freelance and now focuses heavily on recreational riders. His aim is to please the likes of you and me.

'Hello James,' Phil says to a mildly perspiring me after negotiating Mancunian traffic. 'I'll start by saying an expert is someone who's made a lot of mistakes. I've made a lot of mistakes.' And nice to meet you, Phil. I'm presuming you learned from them.

He continues, 'Also be aware that this'll differ to an elite set-up as presumably your goals aren't the same as theirs?' Bit presumptuous but yes. 'Firstly, we'll understand your goals and then work through your history of injury and cycling. We'll then assess your current bike set-up, analyse your saddle, look at footwear and maybe make some changes. But if we do, there's one thing I always say: I don't change anyone's position. You do. If you don't understand why these things are happening and why I'd recommend them, they won't happen.

'So, what's the aim of today?' Phil asks. For elites, this might be maximising sustainable power output or reducing drag on a time trial bike by a nudge of the elbow position. It's all about refining their slipstreamed selves. For me, though, it was about something else. 'I'm increasing mileage,' I reply. 'I'm 45. To me, that means I need to be in a position that reduces my chances of injury.' I then tell Phil about a hot spot in my right foot that warms up on rides over an hour. It ties in with a weird clawing thing in the same foot. Phil scribbles all this down.

'Any breaks?' he asks.

'I fractured my ankle cycling back from the pub.' I know, I know, I know. It was after a Christmas quiz; I'd only had a couple pints but… It happened a few years back but the right ankle does continue to swell up, especially after I've played football. Which naturally leads me to ask Phil the same question I'd put to coach Mosley: 'Can I continue to play football, Phil?'

'It actually might be good for you,' he replies. Unfurl the bunting, pop the party poppers… 'It will have changed the biomechanics of your ankle but football will keep it fairly strong and mobile. Football's a good gauge of the health of your ankle because there's so much eccentric force and loading in five-a-side compared to cycling. They could actually work well together.'

'Anything else?' he probes.

'I have skis for feet.'

I remove my shoes and Phil agrees. I inherited my uber-thin hooves from my mum and I suspect this could be the root of the clawing. 'Yes, you certainly have low-volume feet,' Phil says politely. 'If you have a low-volume foot, there are often issues with over-tightening. But there are solutions for that.'

'I also experience pain down the right side of my knee on long runs,' I tell Phil, warming to the injurious theme.

'That's common. The thing is, human beings are asymmetrical. That can cause issues when running, especially on flat terrain. But it can cause problems with cycling too, because cycling's symmetrical. When you run, you can accommodate that difference. You can't do that easily on a bike because the distances are set. But, usually, people naturally find a way to cope. Yes, we might make a few small adjustments but it's very rare anyone needs a huge overhaul.

'One quote I love from one of the best surgeons I ever worked with was, when you hear hooves, what do you think of? A horse. You don't think of a zebra, do you? That's his point. If it looks like something and feels like something and you have the evidence, it is that. Always a chance it could be something else, but miniscule. A headache's more likely to be a headache than a brain tumour.'

To analyse whether I'm a horse or a zebra, Phil says that he is going to analyse me riding. But before then, the Cornishman has me strutting my stuff down his clinical catwalk.

'Yes, I can see why you had iliotibial band [ITB] issues when running as you're ever so slightly externally rotating your foot. That means your toes are out and your heels are in. If you look down, you can see it, more so on your right than left. When you walk, you're not a duck but [there's] definitely a little external rotating. Do you ever get crank rub?'

'My heel does occasionally catch it,' I reply.

'It's not a problem but tells us something about why your ITB is so tight when running. Now stand on your right leg and make a small knee bend, please. Interesting – when you do that, you manage to correct your rotation. I'm looking at your hip, knee and ankle. Now your left. That's much better.'

Phil's game of 'Simon says' continues with me attempting to touch my toes. And to be fair, I don't make a bad stab at it. 'Now sit on the edge of the table and grab the front of your left knee with both hands if you can. Right, roll back and try and lie down. This is called the

Thomas Test and is used to measure flexibility in your hips… Bloody hell, James, you're worse than me.'

Offensive. But interesting. I'd always thought a certain lack of flexibility was down to tight hamstrings from football. Phil suggests otherwise. My hamstrings are actually really good – Phil's words, not mine – but my hip flexors are, well, simply not flexing. It certainly explains my lack of fluidity on the dance floor (though it doesn't explain the lack of co-ordination or awkwardness…) and, according to Phil, it isn't really an issue because cycling is a 2D motion.

That's the static analysis ticked off. Now it is time for what is euphemistically called the dynamic bike fit. But not before I've grabbed a coffee and wandered around Phil's home from home. It's a cyclist's nirvana with analytical tools and cameras everywhere you look. There's also a skeleton and broken-down parts, including a pelvis, to demonstrate the anatomical pressures of cycling. A full range of Park tools hang from the wall to satisfy the bike mechanics out there, while signed and framed yellow jerseys from his time at Team Sky decorate the wall.

The artificial light reflects brightly off something blue in the corner. 'They're the aero shoes Bradley [Wiggins] wore in the team pursuit at the Rio Olympics,' Phil explains, picking one up and plopping it on my lap. 'They're carbon throughout – that's not just the sole but the last [the form around which a shoe is made], too – and cost £2000. Custom bike-shoe expert David Simmons made them. He flew over from the US and showed me how to cast them. That was a hell of lot of responsibility, especially at that price. You cast the rider's feet and then have to "gently" prise their feet out. You do that by placing a metal strip upfront and then slicing it open with a Stanley knife. Mark Cavendish had a pair, too, and let off an almighty "Aaargghhh" when I cast his. He was only joking, though he didn't wear them in the end as it clashed with his Nike sponsorship. But Jason Kenny wore them, Laura Trott [now Kenny] wore them… They all texted in to say they'd never been more connected with the bike.'

I flip the shoe over to reveal a set of cleats recessed into the sole with a BOA closure dial on the underside rather than above like a normal pair. 'That was for aerodynamic purposes,' says Phil. 'But power purposes, too. Some sprinters enjoyed a massive uplift in maximum power. If a sprinter is in a generic shoe, their foot wobbling around even a tiny bit at around 2000 watts can make a huge difference. This equates to an easy 40 watts, which is huge at that level.' Of course, I can neither afford nor justify such expense on a pair of sleek slippers. There are bigger fish to fry, and more affordable ones at that. But it's all fascinating.

With that, Phil finishes clamping my road bike to his Wahoo Kickr turbo trainer – there's a testing jig I could have used if I hadn't had my bike with me – has me sit on it and peppers me with dots. 'These are stickers, which I'll attach the harness to – that talks to the 3D motion-capture system, which talks to the dongle on the laptop, which will give us all the pose and joint angles we need.'

Once I am all hooked up, an avatar of me appears on the screen, along with a load of data. As Phil explains, 'When you're pedalling, anything in green is good while anything in yellow is outside of the norm of the data Retül has collected over years and years of testing. But there might be a very good reason for that and it might not be a bad thing. You're long-legged, whereas someone like [Chris] Boardman is really short in the legs, which is good for time trialling. With you and your legs, you might, for instance, need a larger frame.'

I begin cycling at an easy wattage and Phil starts observing, making notes. He tells me about a chapter in his bestselling bike-fitting book (called *Bike Fit*) that looks at micro-adjustors and macro-absorbers. Micro-adjustors are those people – you know who you are – who change one thing on their bike and notice it immediately. Williams and Bennett alluded to them earlier. 'Ben Swift [Ineos Grenadiers] was like that,' Phil says. 'He once had four Pinarellos, arguing with the mechanics that one saddle height was higher than the other. I leant on one of the bikes and said, is that the one that feels higher? He said yes. That was the one with the newer, firmer saddle. He's [like the] princess and the pea. Then you have macro-absorbers like Geraint Thomas, who once rode the wrong-sized bike for half the Tour de France and didn't even realise.'

I'd say I'm a macro-absorber. But we'll see. Over the course of the next 45 minutes, Phil plays around with my saddle height, saddle setback and saddle nose position. His Poirot-like powers note that despite an 'excellent pedalling action' (*merci*, Phil), my right knee reached the peak of each circle with a jaunty flourish to the right, which is probably down to my frozen hips. Though it could also be down to crank length, meaning I'm too squeezed when one foot is at the 12 o'clock position.

Adjustments are made and many of the sad yellow figures turn to happy green. He recommends narrower handlebars, my 44cm-wide ones leading to an overstretch and potential injury. But he is still slightly concerned about my wayward knee and recommends a gear change.

'Crank length will solve that. You're using a 175mm crank length. That'd be standard issue with your bike. Most larger bikes come with them that length. This is important at every level. Let me give you an example. Three weeks before Wiggins' hour record in 2015, he was using 177.5mm cranks. That's not unusual as he's a tall lad of 190cm. The problem with that was his knees were coming up into the chest and close to his elbows, which was proving uncomfortable. The idea of longer cranks was to maximise power output. But his hips were too closed at the top. We dropped Wiggins from 177.5mm to 170mm and dropped his front end 30mm. He saved drag, rode faster, and this from a man who'd won the Tour de France. I'll give you an analogy. Would you prefer to jump on to this 1.5m-high box or this 4mm-high box 100 times? Either way, I will give you £100. Which would you choose? Crank length will make a demonstrative difference to your cycling comfort.'

Armed with this new knowledge, on my return to Bristol, I seek out 170mm cranks and narrower handlebars. My Fabric saddle had been declared OK after Phil had assessed my pressure points via his Gebiomized pressure system, which is essentially a high-tech saddle cover that measures the parts of my buttocks that apply most pressure on the perch. Another new weapon in my cycling arsenal is a pair of customised insoles that Phil had fashioned for me using a footbed that resembled putty and what looked like a hairdryer but which Phil had reassured me was something he called a 'top-end saddle gun'. The insoles are for my clawing feet.

We were done. I showered, changed out of Lycra and returned to the lab to have another coffee and remember one more thing. 'I've hired a Wattbike that I'm training on. What should I do about crank length?' 'Don't worry,' Phil says. 'They're 170mm so it's all good.

'But there are a few things you need to do. Firstly, a fan is an essential for indoor training but angle it at your saddle. The increased airflow will cool things down and leave things less sweaty, which is important because heavy sweat, sustained pressure on the saddle and high friction is a disastrous recipe for the skin to break down.'

Phil also advises setting a reminder to stand up every five minutes for further perineal relief and recommends I get a small physio ball to work into my stiff hips and loosen them up. 'That should be it,' he signs off. 'I hope you've enjoyed it and it'll prove useful. I'll email you a report including your set-up dimensions in case your bike is nicked.' And with that, my bike, raised saddle and more efficient me cycle back to Manchester Parkway to catch the train back south.

'Guys, best check your sheds and garages,' the WhatsApp read. 'I've just seen two lads cycle out of the street rolling another bike in their hands.' Oh no. Surely not again. We've lived in the same Victorian cottage about 8km from the centre of Bristol for nearly 14 years. It's been great. Apart from the bike crime. We've had countless bikes stolen, both at home and in Bristol. It's upsetting, making you and your family feel vulnerable. But one of the recent events was almost comical as the brazen bike gangsters unscrewed the shed door, neatly placed it against our crumbling pennant-stone wall, broke the bike locks and rode away.

The message from the WhatsApp group stirred up all those bad memories. I looked out to darkness and saw our garage door had been prised open like a tin of tuna.

'I don't believe it,' I told my wife. 'Four bikes stolen.' Gone are our mountain bikes, a gravel bike and, most annoyingly for this mission, the road bike I'd had measured up in Manchester. We were all shaken. And it went further: it really was the final straw and we put our house on the market soon after.

We're clearly not the only ones suffering from bike crime. According to the Crime Survey for England and Wales victimisation survey, there were an estimated 288,000 incidents of bike theft between April 2017 and March 2018. From my experience, this is an underestimate, with many victims not bothering to inform the police or insurance companies.

This time, I followed the well-practised routine of informing the police, who always reply that they simply didn't have the resources to investigate. It wasn't always thus. When we first had bikes stolen around 13 years ago, they came around, guiding us to what do next and offering a crumb of comfort during an unsettled period. (Though clearly the guidance wasn't failproof!) That changed, presumably as police cuts took hold and bike crime shot up. Now, I simply phoned to take note of a crime reference number.

I then reported my bike stolen on www.stolen-bikes.co.uk. This is a useful website that searches bike adverts across all the major UK classifieds, including Gumtree and eBay. Sadly, the quartet of bikes failed to pop up, though my mate had more success, having his stolen fixie returned four months after it had been nicked. Not liking what they saw, the thieves had dumped it in a woods near his garden. Fussy devils.

It's why I'd implore anyone to insure their bike(s), whether it's via a bike-specific insurer like Yellow Jersey or Laka, or doing what I normally do and topping up home insurance with bike-specific add-ons, including covering bikes away from home. If you buy a new bike, register it on the national cycle database at www.bikeregister.com. Here, you input your bike's details, upload a photo and, more importantly, add your bike's frame number. Your bike's registration number is the swiftest way to retrieve your bike if it's found. It also does no harm when it comes to that insurance claim.

And go lock crazy. I now use Litelok, which is a gold-standard lock and is my on-the-fly option. For home security, our Alcatraz also uses Kryptonite's New York lock that's forged from 16mm-hardened steel.

It's an emotional hit. And a professional one. I've gone from myriad bicycle options to none, aside from a cyclo-cross frame with broken wheels hanging from beams in the garage. It beats me why said thieves didn't take that one…

The professionals aren't immune to bike crime, either, with Trek–Segafredo's women's team twice having bikes stolen when racing in the UK in 2022, amounting to a loss of around £50,000 worth of equipment. Israel Cycling Academy had 17 bikes stolen after their truck was broken into. Chapeau to Romanian police, who recovered 21 of the 22 Italian national team bikes that had been nicked from the hotel car park while the team were competing in the 2021 UCI Track World Cycling Championships in Roubaix, France. Unlike me, though, the pros at least have spares and can instantly replace missing kit.

For now, there is a sticking plaster solution of sorts until I sort out some new wheels. I've hired a Wattbike, which will take pride of place in the kitchen. Everyone in the household, as you can imagine, is delighted with our new addition. As it's winter, cold and generally dark, I won't miss outdoor riding too much. Mosley's plan links to Zwift, meaning the prescribed sessions can be followed virtually, any changes in power reflected on the screen. It's all rather nifty and fine for the midweek shorter, more intense sessions, and I'm quickly into the swing of early morning indoor workouts with the goal of July's L'Étape du Tour at the front, centre and back of my mind. 'Build the base, grow my FTP' is my new mantra. But the longer Sunday ride could become a little monotonous. I'll have to come up with a solution for that, and rather fast.

3

Crossover to Road

T-minus five and a half months

Mud, glorious mud. Pigs wallow in it and tyres slip on it. Or grip in it, depending on knobbles, power output and torque. That's right, it's January 2022 and I'm in Ardingly. I've headed to West Sussex for the British National Cyclo-Cross Championships, held this year at the South of England Showground.

What's to know about Ardingly, pronounced Ardin-lie? Well, journalist Jon Snow, the skyscraper of a newsreader, was born here, and according to Wikipedia, it also runs a 'low-level frequency bus service to the nearby towns of Haywards Heath and Crawley'.

I'm unsure what low level is, but low, high or moderate, I've foregone the local transport network in favour of a brisk 9.7km country walk from my overnight abode in leafy Haywards Heath. It's early on Sunday. I'd arrived the previous afternoon after a four-hour train journey from Bristol, the aim being to catch Haywards Heath Town FC in the Isthmian League South East division. I've grown to love watching non-league football thanks to my author pal Nige Tassell, seeing the appeal of a good standard of football for a fiver, regular battles in the dugout, all the while being able to wander the entire ground. The crowds are never huge. But they were even thinner on my drenched Saturday arrival as the referee had called the match off following 24 hours of incessant rain.

But by Sunday, it's now a winter's morning that has 'crisp' coursing through its frozen veins, a keen but tepid sun sending temperatures fluctuating between visible breath and numb fingertips. I've packed my standard journalistic fare into my reliable, stoical but frayed Thule rucksack: laptop, spare clothes, digital voice recorder, notepad, bottle of water, energy bar and peanuts.

Why am I wading through this mud pit when the likes of Egan Bernal and Primož Roglič make their names and fortunes – both earn around £5 million a year – on tarmac? Wouldn't it be more prudent to head to Alicante to spend a week with Tour phenomenon Tadej Pogačar on a winter's training camp? (OK, I had tried that one but Covid said no.)

The reason is thus: every year since 2014, every cyclo-cross world champion has been, or has become, a star of the road. So, since my main goal is to complete a stage of the Tour de France, and in my highly diluted way to mimic the seasonal timeline of the pros, there's a double hit of inspiration to be had by attending. In 2014, Czech rider Zdeněk Štybar, who competes on the WorldTour for Belgian outfit Quick-Step, pipped cyclo-cross legend Sven Nys to the crown. Nys was a bona fide crosser, winning 50 World Cups and two world titles. But his 2013 victory would prove to be the last time a pure cyclo-cross rider would win the men's title. Since Štybar, between 2015 and 2021, the event was dominated by Dutchman Mathieu van der Poel and Belgian Wout van Aert, who won seven times between them, van der Poel edging things four to three.

Both riders are now arguably the biggest names in road cycling. Cycling chameleon van der Poel had flirted with road while excelling at not only cyclo-cross but also mountain biking. But in 2019, he made the decision to focus more on the road. Much hype surrounded this switch, though he still races cross, as beyond his off-road prowess, his maternal grandfather was French cyclist Raymond Poulidor, who won the Vuelta a España in 1964. However, the French didn't love Raymond for his success. Their eternal *amour* derived from defeat, Poulidor finishing runner-up at the Tour de France three times and in third place a further five times. Van der Poel's father, Adri, had road pedigree, too, winning the Dutch National Championships six times and racking up several classic successes plus two stage victories at the Tour. He also won the Cyclo-cross World Championships in 1996.

Van der Poel's family lineage, palmarès and good looks diverted the attention from Slovak Peter Sagan and on to the Dutchman for the 2019 spring classic season. Could this potent mix of nature being nurtured light up the grey northern European one-dayers? Was there any doubt? At Amstel Gold Race, an annual one-day classic held in the province of Limburg, the Netherlands, where the peloton cover over 260km in just shy of seven hours, van der Poel recorded what Eurosport commentator Rob Hatch described as, 'One of the most incredible wins you're ever likely to see in the history of professional cycling.'

With a 10-man breakaway over a minute up the road, van der Poel went on the attack around 40km from the finish on the punchy Gulperberg climb. The out-of-the saddle effort had cyclo-cross stamped all over it. And naivety, as he soon drifted back to the chasing peloton. It seemed the inexperienced road rider had received a lesson in race strategy.

Au contraire. Van der Poel dug deep, turning a minute's disadvantage into a sprinkling of seconds over the last 10km. That digging reached oil-discovery status come the final sprint when, despite his exertions, he slungshot off leader Jakob Fuglsang's wheel for an incredible and unlikely victory.

A new road star had arrived, van der Poel's reputation enhanced further by wins at the Tour of Flanders and Strade Bianche, plus a stage victory at the 2021 Tour de France that would see him wear the sacred yellow jersey for six days. His grandfather would have been proud.

Van Aert's own achievements at Jumbo–Visma – including numerous Tour stage wins, plus success at one-day classics Milan–San Remo, Strade Bianche, Gent–Wevelgem and Amstel Gold Race – had coaches and pundits questioning their training dogma, dissecting why these athletes who spent much of their winter competing in mud were so strong come the road.

'I can but speculate but I feel there are many reasons.' The words there of Yorkshireman Alex Rhodes. I accosted Rhodes in the Ardingly quagmire. He'd compete in the professional race later that day, his first at elite national championships level, but would be pulled out due to the 80 per cent rule. We'll come back to that later. He's a former professional triathlete, lives for endurance sport and is currently being encouraged to shimmy along by his wife and baby. But he's oblivious – he just loves cycling. 'Firstly, it's great for improving your handling on the road. You've got tight, technical turns and you want to take those at speed to keep on the wheel of the guy in front. You're constantly having to play around with your weight and position on the saddle, as it takes quite an effort to just remain upright.

'Then there's the relentless power output,' Rhodes continues. 'On a muddy course like this, there's no freewheeling – you've just got to keep pedalling and pedalling and...'

These physiological demands are extreme. While the racing 'only' consumes an hour compared to a road stage that can roll on for five to six hours, the intensity's all-out. Road, on the other hand, is a longer, lower-intensity effort around the French countryside before a final intense burst. How extreme cyclo-cross is was highlighted by a 2017 study in the open journal *Sports and Exercise Medicine*[4]. A team led by Ryanne Carmichael, associate professor of exercise and sports physiology at Plymouth State University, USA, had eight experienced crossers take part in both a lab test and a cyclo-cross race.

In the lab, they pedalled to exhaustion on a cycle ergometer, the researchers measuring a number of metrics, including lactate production at the increasing intensities. I go into detail about the impact of this perceived physiological devil in Chapter 4. For now, it's enough to know that the fitter you are, the higher your power output while keeping these lactate levels low. In Carmichael's study, heart rate intensities were categorised as low, medium and high – like Ardingly's bus service – where low equates to lactate levels of 2mmol/litre or under, up to high, at 4mmol/l or over.

The octet of lab rats then scuttled over to a 2.7km lapped course on varied terrain including grass, pavement and barriers and went hell for race leather over an hour. 'Subjects had an average heart rate of 170.8 beats per minute [bpm] and a maximum of 177.8bpm,' wrote

Carmichael. 'The percentage of time in low, medium and high zones was 0.3, 6.1 and 93.6 per cent, respectively.'

'Cyclo-cross racing is performed at a higher intensity than road, criterium or mountain-bike racing,' Carmichael concluded. 'The time spent in the high zone in the current study [93.6 per cent] suggests that the sport requires a significant contribution from the anaerobic energy systems.'

In short, integrate winter cyclo-cross into your plan and, come the road season, once you've sprayed off the detritus, you'll be physically primed and your competitive synapses will be glowing. It's not solely the preserve of the elites, of course, as it's on the radar for amateurs like me. But not today. Today, I'm here to watch and learn from the fastest in the sport.

They're certainly sizzling along in the junior men's race, which has just started on this bright and breezy Sunday morn, following Ella Maclean-Howell's stunning victory in the junior women's race. The start of the snaky circuit is about the only stretch that doesn't require waders. And don't the testosterone-fuelled youths know it, charging along the gravel and towards the first corner, where I'm stationed with the abandon of Pamplona bulls. The frenzied herd seek prime position to negotiate the first turn incident-free, but to sighs and gasps from the cornered crowd, one rider hits the deck. It's the only time in the race when he'd have preferred mud.

Those who remain upright then swiftly have speed scrubbed out by churned-up terrain and a sandpit before shifting up a gear over a temporary wooden bridge and then weaving their way to what the programme notes simply term 'steep banks'. 'Mud-spattered Eiger' might have been more appropriate. The course digs down, then up and around, the riders defying gravity and the sucking of soil much to the delight of the surprisingly large crowd, who show their appreciation with a clanging of the cowbells – a ritual picked up from Belgium, where the popularity of cyclo-cross is akin to Premier League football in the UK.

Belgium is the sport's heartland and would host five of the 15 World Cup rounds in the 2021–2022 season. Crowds turn out in their tens of thousands to cheer on their heroes while drinking copious amounts of 8% beer against the backdrop of a banging Europop soundtrack. Here in Ardingly, they've looked to replicate the Belgian disco, albeit, befitting the weekend's deluge, in watered-down form. Despite some banging beats, the rave tent's more like a grave tent, the duo of attendees preferring to recline on fold-up chairs over fist pumping and head swinging. Still, locals Bedlam Brewery are doing a swift trade. As is the *frites* stall, the queue for which is either down to exquisite cuisine or the nominal food stands. Either way, despite the grave tent, the celebratory atmosphere is an appreciated tonic to the Covid blues of the past couple of years.

After 40 minutes of high-octane racing, Joseph Smith wins, with Ben Askey second and Max Greensill third. There's an hour's break until the next championship race, the senior and under-23 women's elite, so I purchase an Americano from Sussex Coffee Trucks and take in part of the 150-acre showground. Its roots are agricultural, with June's South of England Show its flagship event. Come the summer, this is the place to learn about livestock, sample sheep shearing and enjoy the Young Farmers' Club doing battle for a year's bragging rights at the tug-of-war competition.

The perma-rural aroma's temporarily replaced by the tang of petroleum, the racers applying litres of winter-specific wet lube to fend off the muck. There's a 'sand school' for equestrian fans at the South of England Show, which for this weekend doubles as a sandpit, and next to that is the car park that for this weekend is being used as a caravan park. It's packed with the competitors' mobile homes and trailers with awnings marking out further land for last-minute tweaks. Tyres are inflated and then deflated, riders warm up upon rollers and eyewear is steamed and polished.

It's a colourful, at times garish, spectacle with many of the race suits emblazoned with sponsors seeking on-the-fly visibility. The cyclo-cross bikes are a classier affair, the vibrant but more selective colour palette befitting bikes that can cost up to 10 grand. From a distance, they're road bikes but edge closer and the subtle differences become more marked and more important. First, there are the obvious – tyres, which are wider and knobbly – then there's the less obvious, like geometry, gears, often tougher frames and often shorn of bottle cages to allow the riders to carry the bikes. The sight of bikes being carried is a common one today because of the mud-spattered fields, but the courses also generally include barriers and other obstacles that require riders to dismount and transport their steeds at a run. Like Ardingly, many courses also comprise a mix of pavement, gravel, grass and sand, and include hills, flat sections and off-camber portions.

This run element drew attention to Ineos Grenadiers' Tom Pidcock at the start of 2021 when he posted on Strava a 5km training run time of 13 minutes and 25 seconds (he wasn't carrying a bike at the time!). He later posted on social media, 'Maybe running is the sport for me.' It would seem so as this time was only five seconds shy of the British record over that distance, set by Marc Scott in August 2020. As it transpired, though, either the GPS was out or there had been some user error and in fact the time wasn't quite correct. Either way, Pidcock's run speed is certainly impressive, and helps in cyclo-cross.

As I continue to stroll around the showground, one bike in particular glitters in the winter sun. It's a pearlescent purple with the brand Scott picked out in bright yellow on the top tube. It's pristine and beautiful and I wish it were mine. (I love a pearlescent colourway and remember with fondness a steel Peugeot my parents treated me to when I was young.) The bike belongs to the Peak District's Nick Craig. My experience of cyclo-cross is nominal, though growing, but I've heard of Craig. Born in 1969 in Stockport, he has won countless national championships and is a legend of the sport.

'OK to grab a word, Nick?' I ask. 'Best not as I'm racing in the elite race soon. Later,' he replies. The elite race?! Craig is 51 and competed in the downpour 24 hours earlier, winning the 50–54 age category in a time of 43.13 minutes. The races tend to be 40 or 60 minutes long and the faster riders will complete more laps, with commissaires or timing chips keeping a track of who is where. In today's elite races, the 80 per cent rule is implemented, whereby any rider whose lap time is 80 per cent off the leader's lap time is pulled from the race, which will be the case for Alex Rhodes. Craig, despite his half century and racing a day earlier, will be there.

Time passes in a flurry of chocolate cake and coffee, and cheers echo around the showground as Harriet Harnden storms to the women's elite title. In the process, the 21-year-old Trek Factory Racing cyclo-cross star wins the under-23 category, too.

I flick through my programme and see it's the men's elite event up next. It's the final race of the weekend and the most eagerly awaited as Pidcock's down on the starting list. However, he has withdrawn at the last minute. It's a shame for the crowd and the organisers, Crawley Wheelers, who'd capitalised on Pidcock's growing profile by using a photo of a young Pidcock at a previous national championships on the cover of the programme. Still, it doesn't seem to have affected the party atmosphere as inflatable dinosaurs merrily make their way past elite riders warming up on rollers. Even the grave tent has more of a rave feel about it now and I'm smiling in the winter's sun. I really didn't realise it would be such a proper sporting event, which is incredibly patronising but is meant as high praise for the Wheelers and all who've made this such a wonderful place to be on a Sunday in January. (I might not have said that if I'd attended 24 hours earlier in the deluge, of course.)

With no Pidcock, Cameron Mason of Trinity Racing – Pidcock's former team – is installed as pre-race favourite after a strong season thus far, including under-23 victory in the Dendermonde leg of the UCI Cyclo-cross World Cup. Gateshead rider Thomas Mein's also being talked about as a contender.

I head to the far corner, where the crowds are at their densest, the atmosphere is at its liveliest and the mud is at its thickest. The steep banks have already gone down in cyclo-cross folklore and the weekend's not yet complete. But before I reach the banks of doom, cheering's replaced by humming. And a gushing sound. Against the bright sun and gradient of the hill, its source remains a mystery, until the brow is reached and all is revealed: myriad bikes are being jet-washed by armies of soaked individuals. Six large water tanks sit upon wooden crates from which water-carriers (cleaners) fill their vessels. It's even muddier than the steep banks section and is metaphorically the pits. Literally, too, as it transpires.

'Yes, this is the pit area,' explains Grant Fraser, who is brandishing his jet wash like a particularly dedicated paintballer. Fraser is a rider himself but is here in support of rider Danny Clark. 'Danny will come through here every lap or two and we'll swap bikes. We'll then clean up his dirty one for his next pit stop. It's a common tactic when conditions are like they are today. When it's really muddy, your drivetrain [gears, cassette and chain] fills up with crap. That makes things less efficient and weighs you down. A clean bike makes a world of difference.'

Fraser laments his jet washer as it's battery operated and less powerful than the humming petrol ones. But he's doing his bit for the environment. And for Clarke's performance, since he finishes a respectable 46th in a competitive field of 73 starters. Craig comes in an incredible 12th, the 53-year-old just behind 21-year-olds Jenson Young and Joe Coukham in 10th and 11th, respectively. But the winner is Mein, who edges out Mason by four seconds for his first senior national title.

'It was such an epic battle with Mason from start to finish,' Mein said after the race. 'It took everything I had to beat him.' Mein would continue to race cyclo-cross into February before swapping knobblies for slicks and racing for his British Continental team, WiV SunGod.

The crowds begin to disperse while the jet washes continue to wipe away the muddy memories of recent events. I return to the car park/ caravan park and spot a slightly dirtier version of Craig's pearlescent purple beauty. 'OK to chat now, Nick?' 'Of course.'

And chat we do. It turns out that Nick Craig is as generous with interviews as he is brutal to his opposition, and epitomises the warm, inclusive community that every winter congregates on mud. I start by congratulating Nick on his 12th in the elite race and check in on the old man's condition.

'Strangely, racing the Saturday clears away the cobwebs. Sven Nys was like that. He'd generally get stronger through the weekend. That said, there are a lot of good over-50s so I can't rest on my laurels.

But I guess I'm still driven. I remember sitting in a hotel with Tom [Pidcock] a couple of years ago. His mechanic was really good at motivating Tom and said, "Right, tomorrow, Tom, what we need to do is clear the pits. You know how busy the pits are. There'll be 120 riders with 120 pit crews and all the water and stuff. Each time you come within 80 per cent of any of those riders, they'll be thrown out of the race as the 80 per cent rule applies. Tom looks at me and says, "I'm going to get you pulled." I said you cheeky shit, there is no way.

'The wife thought it was hilarious. She was helping out in the pits and said they're getting really quiet. I said, have you enough water [to clean my bike]? She said, "Don't worry, I won't need some soon". She was right as Tom got us but I was one of the last to be pulled.'

It was a rare occurrence. Craig's the most celebrated cyclo-cross star on the British scene, though he mountain biked for Great Britain at the 2000 Sydney Olympics. He also rode the Tour of Mallorca in 2004, but it's cyclo-cross where his heart lies. He's ridden the northern winter leagues for years, winning the celebrated Three Peaks race for the first time in 1991. 'I didn't know it when I was growing up but my Dad won it in 1963 in only its third edition. That was nice.'

I asked Craig how long he'll continue to race for. 'My wife says that when you look like you're letting yourself down – that means snot hanging from your nose, dribbling from your face and looking old – you're not doing it, you're done. But not yet.'

Certainly not from his Ardingly showing. Craig's technique stood out. He had an upright, controlled manner that looked effortless. Or at least efficient. His body remained stiller than my tight hips while his legs flowed at a high cadence.

'Nothing feels better than beating someone who's fitter and stronger than you. But you can do that in cyclo-cross on the technical and tactical side. I grew up without gear indexing; without fancy stuff. When I stroke the pedals in those circles, it's because I grew up without fancy electric groupsets. You become more in tune with gear changes and aspects like that.

'In the race just gone, I went past a guy in his mid-30s. I'm not into watts but this guy's average power is around 400 watts constantly.

After, I said to him you do realise I was sat behind you on one of the long drags to the tech area. He was pushing on those pedals and putting out huge watts. But in the mud, he wasn't getting much back from it. So, I noticed that if I backed off a bit and took it a little easier, I'd go the same speed as him. So, I had a rest. When I went past him, I cracked him and didn't see him again. It's an example of where you put your power out, how you put your power out and how to read the race situation… If you're not going to maintain grip, the more power you put down, the more your wheels are going to slide and less is transmitted to the ground. I guess I'm efficient.'

I make a mental note of this efficiency as it's not just applicable to the dirty world of cyclo-cross. OK, ultimately L'Étape du Tour will be on the smoothest terrain you can expect anywhere – apparently this is because the French use a finer grain of tarmac than here in the UK as parts are drier – but being efficient over 100 miles, on any terrain but especially climbing 5000 very long metres, will be key to thriving, surviving or receiving a damn good hiding.

There are many ways to be efficient on the bike, both gear-wise and physically. One method that efficiently feeds back to performance on- and off-road is pedalling technique. The French call the art of perfect pedalling 'souplesse'. Only the French would create a term that made pedalling sound delicious. Visually, a rider with souplesse gives the appearance of generating effortless speed. Practically, it means pedalling in circles. I'd noticed on the Wattbike I'd hired that there's a data field on the Wattbike app that assesses pedal technique. It's a computer-generated diagram that can be broadly broken down into three shapes: the figure-of-eight, the peanut and the sausage. A figure-of-eight shows that the cyclist is losing pedal momentum on the transition from one leg to the next; the peanut shape is better but still shows some loss of momentum; the sausage is elite level, showing strong momentum throughout. For a man who loves peanuts, I was very pleased to say I'd naturally started in the peanut position. I might not be generating a huge power output but what I was putting out was ticked off rather efficiently. Let's hope that my peanut pedalling would pay dividends in both cyclo-cross and on the road.

Anyway, I digress. Back to that man Craig, whose tactical nous was spotted by British Cycling, for whom he worked between 2004 and 2005. 'I was a technical coach and remember saying to Dave Brailsford that we could replicate the pathway from track to road for cyclo-cross to road. My argument was that the facility of cyclo-cross was a safer environment than a velodrome for young kids and you can ride everywhere. But cyclo-cross isn't on the Olympic schedule and British Cycling is a medal factory, so it never took off.'

Maybe not formally, but recent times have seen many young off-road riders graduate to the WorldTour road circuit, including Ben Turner and Pidcock, who both now race for Ineos Grenadiers, though Craig's first experience of Britain's great new road hope was ironically on the track. 'I remember seeing Tom when he was 16. I was athlete mentor for the Sainsbury's School Games, which was track-based in the Manchester Velodrome. I said I haven't got a track background but they just wanted someone who's experienced the Olympic village and ridden at a good level.

'Turner was there, too, and they were all riding for Yorkshire. I remember watching the team pursuit on the last day and there was this scrawny kid with hardly any muscle in a pink skinsuit that didn't really fit him – Yorkshire had pink for some reason. Well, I went home that night and said to my wife Sarah, and Charlie and Thomas, "I've just seen the next Bradley Wiggins". Again, it was the way he pedalled. He looked so efficient and smooth, and generated power and speed from a body that didn't look capable.'

Charlie and Thomas are Sarah and Nick's sons. Sadly, Charlie died in January 2017. The 15-year-old went to sleep and never woke up. An inquest 12 months later determined that he'd had a heart attack. 'He was a natural and had just won the national series, beating Ben Tulett and Lewis Askey, who both now race on the WorldTour. He also lost in a sprint finish with Ben at the National Champs just two weeks before we lost him. I remember that was one he wanted to win because his older brother, Thomas, had won it.

'His older brother won a fair few races and also rode the Mountain Bike Worlds in Andorra. He then retired as he wanted to get his degree. Which was great. We were never pushy parents. For us, it's about enjoyment. About being good sports people and good people.'

Nick's voice breaks slightly. He's clearly a good man. A strong man. With an equally strong partner in Sarah. 'We could have walked away from all of it but we decided to do the opposite because of this community, which is our extended family. It's different to road racing. People are always surprised just how friendly it is. We'll never know what Charlie's future would have held but his memory lives on.'

Nick and Sarah set up Ride for Charlie (www.rideforcharlie.com) to support young off-road cyclists. 'We were hit by the pandemic but the funds are still healthy. We have four teams going to the youth worlds in August after my wife managed to secure support from the Rapha Foundation.'

Nick and I go our separate ways but this day will stay with me forever. It's been one of the greatest sporting events I've ever had the pleasure to attend, where the milk of human kindness is positively overflowing. I've also gained ideas to integrate into my own performance – that handling, tactical acumen and pacing are essential to off-road speed. This triumvirate of skills will transfer nicely to the road and my Étape du Tour challenge. Soon, I vow, I will make my debut cyclo-cross appearance. I mean, how hard can it be?

Angels are portrayed as cherub-like figures with pure-white wings and a glowing halo. That's wrong. I've seen one. His face was youngish but ageing rapidly due to having two children, and temporarily marked each and every day by grime. This angel was stick thin, loves drum and bass, and can miraculously mend battered cyclo-cross wheels at a day's notice for an upcoming cyclo-cross practice session. This angel is Greg 'Bomber' Lancaster of Bomber Bikeworks on the fringes of Bristol.

After returning inspired from Ardingly, I'd signed up for the ShamXross cyclo-cross race in Keynsham, just between Bristol and Bath, taking place on the last weekend of January. The problem was that those naughty burglars had accidentally left me with only a long-disused frame, bars and spoke-less wheels. A strange axle system – one was thru-axle, one quick-release – meant replacement wheels weren't an option. I'd then seen that the Sham organisers were hosting a practice session a week before the race, so, in light of my cyclo-cross history – zero (I'd used my broken cyclo-cross bike for every ride imaginable apart from cyclo-cross!) – I thought it wise to sign up to that too.

'But will a hired mountain bike be OK?' I emailed co-organiser Heidi Blunden of Parallel Coaching? 'Absolutely fine,' Blunden replied. 'You'll have a blast.' I might look a little out of place, I thought, but it's all for the greater good: honing my fitness and biking skills for the Alpine mountain fest that is L'Étape du Tour. Well, as it transpired, the Angelic Bomber rebuilt my hoops in record time, meaning the Keynsham Chocolate Quarters, once home to Cadbury's but now playing fields plus a luxury retirement village, office space and bar, would welcome me and my lithe cross bike instead of my rented mountain heavyweight.

As in Sussex, I'm welcomed by the cross community beneath clear blue skies, though it's rather chilly at 2°C, but with two hours' coaching and riding ahead, I have no fears of not heating up on this Saturday morning. What's more, I'm already pretty warm after carrying two fence panels home first thing in an effort to patch up our garden and sell our house. Today's session is hosted by Blunden and course designer Kev Brewer. Brewer's been busy as the following week's parcours has already been pegged out. Disappointingly, this morning's focus will be on the pitchy, hilly bit rather than the majority of the route that's flat. Sadists.

Today's crowd is a reassuring mix. Many wear club tops, whether it's the red of Clevedon or the orange and blue of Bristol CX; others are in off-the-peg numbers, like my Rapha jacket, which had been my sister's way of giving me a gentle Étape kick up the behind for Christmas. I'm hoping the array of customised clothing is a sign of keenness but not the excellence I might associate with club disciples. Anyway, that's out of my control and not something to worry about. There are much more pressing matters ahead.

We start easy, weaving in and out of cones. Heidi and Kev then throw in the extra skill of mounting and dismounting. Now, I've done a fair few Olympic-distance triathlons in the past, albeit not that swiftly. Still, I'm incredibly static for the first few hop-offs and hop-ons before relatively finding my stride. I do note, however, something I had noticed at Ardingly – that most of the attendees don't have bottle cages screwed to their frames. That space is needed so you can grip on and lug your steed during the run sections.

'Right, time for the banked training,' announces Blunden. From afar, the pitch beneath the leafless trees looks imperceptible. Edge closer and it seems you need crampons. OK, I'm exaggerating, but for such a short stretch, it looks incredibly testing. 'Grip is all important here,' says Kev. 'Good tyres will help.'

Aha, that's a win. At Ardingly, I'd got talking to Rory Hitchens of Sussex-based distributors Upgrade Bikes. Hitchens has been in the industry since John Boyd Dunlop's time and knows everyone and everything about cycling gear. He was at the Nationals both out of his love of the sport, but also with his Challenge Tires hat on, who are one of their key brands. I'd got talking to Rory about tyres … for 30 minutes. Rory can chat. But usefully so.

'What Challenge has done, which is particularly relevant in cross, is create a much more supple sidewall. The tyre moves and flexes. If you imagine a bit of cloth, it's very easy to move that cloth. If you fill that cloth with rubber, it's stiffer and harder to bend. So, a higher thread count in the sidewall casing and a softer, supple sidewall where the tread's doing the work and is allowed to deform…

'Basically, that allows the tyre to squish flatter on every single bump. Grip's improved. When you're racing in the winter, when you have a lot of mud like we have here, you're looking for tread patterns that cut through the mud to the firmer ground beneath. If you have a bigger tyre like on a mountain bike, you're going to be picking up a lot of mud, which weighs the bike down. So key is keeping a light weight.'

I bagged a set of Challenge Grifo tyres, which Rory informed me are good all-rounders. He also gave me some free advice. 'If you

have the power, a low cadence might actually give you more grip.'
Damn – the main technique I thought I knew was that a high cadence
is needed to overcome the mud. 'Not always. You could spin out in
too low a gear, like mountain biking. Same on a steep climb. Too low
a gear and you could lose grip. Sometimes, if you can keep torque
high and cadence low, you'll enjoy more grip as [you] won't slip on a
root that's coming out from beneath you.'

Rory's advice spins around my head as I face the bank. One go, two
goes, three goes… Nope, I cannot ascend on that mud at that gradient
and remain on the bike. In a timely episode of pathetic fallacy, grey
clouds fill the once blue sky, which perversely seems to illuminate
the grey pylons. 'Don't worry, it'll come,' says Kev. I appreciate your
optimism, Kev.

The practice route is extended to take in further banking, which
not only requires power and grip, but balance, too, as it's a sharp left
camber. I've mountain biked for a few years but this is well beyond my
comfort zone. The lactic acid's building and some of the techniques
needed are next-level, certainly for my current skillset. But on we go.
Practice makes perfect and all that. Through the streams of sweat
and frustration, it's actually damn enjoyable, and I'm beginning to see
why those top roadies are benefitting from a winter spent doing cross.
It naturally has a physicality about it that's achievable on the road
but in a more formalised manner. And the techniques of handling,
of maintaining balance, of gear selection, of cadence selection, well,
they're simply not the norm on an everyday road ride.

I'm shattered but immensely pleased that I shelled out £15 for a real
insight into the race that will take place one week later. Heidi and Kev
have been great, and Heidi finishes things off by running through what
I could plunder for the race: 'The banked section is one third of the
course. The way you approach it can make or break your race; think
about your strengths and exploit them. For example, if you're a good
runner then you may be faster on some parts of the banked session off
the bike than on it. Think momentum! Keep your bike moving along
whether you're riding or running. Smooth riders are fast riders. There's
no "right way". Devise a plan that works for you. This is different for

everyone. Decide early and commit to it. Things can change every lap so be adaptable. Ride and/or run different line choices. By doing this, you'll have different options available in different scenarios. For example, on the first lap when everyone is bunched up.'

The first thing I'll do is drop tyre pressure. The Angelic Bomber had pumped up my Challengers for everyday use and I failed to deflate them before the session. Rory, at hearty length, had told me that it's crucial to find the balance point between tyre pressure and your tread pattern so you secure the best grip. When it's muddy, as in Ardingly and today in Keynsham, you want to go as low as you can get away with.

'Yesterday, Nick Craig was running 17psi pressure in a small-volume tyre,' he said. 'And he knows what he's doing.' Everyone in cyclo-cross knows that man Craig.

I'm just about to ride back to the car when Kev directs us all to the picnic table beneath the gazebo that's doubling as race HQ. 'Take one of these,' he says. 'My wife made them. She's very creative.' She certainly is. I pick up the A4 sheet that's been neatly folded, with SX circled on the cover – it's shorthand for ShamXross – and entitled 'Race Prep Zine 2022'. Back in the warmth of the car, I unfold the paper to reveal seven steps to race success:

1 NOW
Enter race online
BUY or borrow those new mud tyres
CHECK your kit
What else do you need to repair, fix, replace? Buy parts NOW!

2 T-2 weeks
Set-up = test tubeless tyres and test them! Ride them hard at low pressure and race pace and check they don't burp.

3 T-1 week
Polish and wax frame = stops mud sticking! Check weather and adjust kit list. Wash and check kit. Read event guide (check email). Find lucky socks.

4 Race-1 day

Pack kit! Skinsuit, warm-up tights, shoes and studs, race socks, helmet, gloves, two base layers, warm jacket, waterproof puffer jacket, Dry Robe, sponsor's gilet, bobble hat, sunglasses, leg warm-up balm, spare safety pins, Vicks, two bikes, rollers, pre-race snack, pre-race carb drink, post-race protein shake and bar, race licence, debit card, mask and alcohol gel. ~~Race bottle~~ never [because that's not only added weight but impedes carrying your bike].

5 Race day

Arrive on time and sign on; collect race number and chip; do sighting lap – be alert! Where do you/other riders struggle? Adjust tyre pressures on both bikes to match course conditions. Take spare bike to pits; warm up on rollers; don't miss gridding! Hydrate. Ride like the wind and have fun. Return race number and chip.

6 Race evening

Clean bikes. Clean now, tomorrow = concrete; wash your kit now! What went well? Need to remember for next time? Write it down!

7 Race+1 day

Check lap times; check bike and kit for damage; do yoga; look for next race; check ShamXross website for photos.

It's brilliant and beautiful, epitomising the community spirit of this wonderful sport. How much of it I'll follow in the upcoming week during which work looks flat out is debatable. But I definitely know I won't be ticking off the cleaning-bike aspect of number six!

Sunday, 30 January 2022 – the day of my race – proved something of a ground-breaking day for the world of cyclo-cross. As commentator Rob Hatch said, 'Fans want something and he delivers. What a cyclo-cross rider he is.' Yes, a British man had achieved something the home nation had long been waiting for. It was a performance of undoubted skill, tactical acumen and pure physical talent. Sadly, I was not the British man... Tom Pidcock, adopting a Superman pose at the finish line, had beaten off the Belgian flotilla to become the first British rider to win the World Cyclo-cross Championships. They were held in Fayetteville, USA, five hours behind GMT, meaning I was washed, dried, early in my pyjamas and watching it on Eurosport after my own cyclo-cross efforts earlier in the day.

We had things in common – a bike, helmet, lungs – but Pidcock clearly cheated by not only riding, cornering, ascending and descending very fast, but running like an Olympian, too. The US course featured the infamous 39 steps, which had to be seen to be believed. Pidcock dismounted, eased his bike on to his shoulder and sprinted up the steps with a biomechanical efficiency and speed that bordered on the obscene. And he did it again and again. I don't know where he'd bagged up and binned his fatigue but he simply didn't tire.

Unlike me. I'd completed my debut cyclo-cross race on the same day and survived but not without enduring an hour's racing where my heart rate averaged 168bpm, which is over 92 per cent of my maximum. Like the week before at the Keynsham practice session, blue skies had provided a stunning backdrop to the hour-long race but it was still chilly. That meant, or so I thought, wearing bib longs, jacket, thick gloves and a base layer. This proved to be a mistake. Despite the near-zero temperatures, when I ride hard, I turn into a fan oven. This became abundantly clear after 10 minutes when sweat flowed down my Rapha-insulated back. I offloaded my gloves but the thermostat was stuck, meaning I had to endure 50 more minutes of high-mercury, high-pain pedalling.

For those first 10 minutes, things went well. But that fanning of the flames was a sign of a poor pacing strategy that saw me melt in the Chocolate Quarters. Those whom I overtook early on returned the disfavour and it wasn't long before the leaders passed me, usually on my right with a loud, 'Right!' I'd also made the error of not knowing myself. I drink a lot on the bike even if it's just a short commute. But seeing no one else with a bottle in their cage, I had dispensed with my sole bottle. I'd told myself it was for ease of carrying the bike, but I had been a sheep following the flock, a thirsty one at that, and would pay for it.

That's when I took a deep breath and focused on me, myself and I, more specifically the process not the end point. This is a technique-heavier discipline than road riding, so you need to pay greater attention to smoother turns on the section of course featuring concentric circles; picture yourself dismounting and mounting while dismounting and mounting over the artificial barriers; and yes, listen to Kev and Heidi's advice of thinking momentum on that damn bank.

Concentrating on these things had a Zen-like effect and, though my heart rate remained high, the haze lifted and I increasingly enjoyed riding around a quagmire in deepest, darkest Keynsham. Pearl Jam bellowed over the speakers and all was increasingly good with the world. The cream on the Jam, however, would be nailing that damn bank without having to put my foot down. And so it happened. I'd approached said bank from what I thought was every conceivable angle but this time, this one time, the tyres, body position and power output came together as one to grip the muddy Everest and reach its approximately 4m peak. 'Keep the torque high and cadence low,' Hitchens had said. 'You'll enjoy more grip.'

And he was right. After an hour's racing, the show was over. It had been exhausting and I can see why in those studies the anaerobic component was so high. Whether you're riding or running on mud, it's draining, every rotation of the wheel or stride encountering much greater rolling resistance than on tarmac. It's what makes it such a devastatingly productive workout, perhaps not one for every day – I felt shattered the next day though my limbs didn't ache – but certainly as part of a rounded off-season programme. Unfortunately, my cyclo-cross taster doubled as the last event of the winter, but I'd enjoyed it and wanted more. For L'Étape du Tour in July, it had given me a physical and psychological nudge. Long term, the cyclo-cross community has a new member. And I'd also just sorted myself a Vitus road bike via Wiggle.

Away from the Keynsham quagmire, I'd continued to spend three or four sessions a week on the Wattbike. These were a hearty mix of sessions for various physiological adaptations. As a sampler and in the words of my TrainingPeaks doctrine: 'sub-threshold, low-cadence efforts to increase cycling-related leg strength with every pedal stroke'; 'MAP [maximal aerobic power] efforts' to, as the name suggests, build aerobic power; 'long aerobic rides for improved fat burning and to boost mitochondria [energy powerhouses in the cells].'

The indoor training was going well, which I'm sure fended off my annual winter chest infection. What's more, road riding upon an actual road bike was also back on the menu thanks to my Wiggle purchase – with my position tweaks from Phil Burt (*see* Chapter 2) – which would be more appetising as spring ticked closer. All in all, things were looking up, as they had to with three huge mountains rapidly appearing on the horizon…

4

The Bloody Secret to Speed

T-minus four months

At the 2022 Tour de France, Tadej Pogačar outsprinted Michael Matthews to victory on stage six from Binche to Longwy. At 219.9km, it marked the longest parcours of the race and finished with a short but steep pitch. One day later, the Slovenian won again in a thrilling battle with eventual winner Jonas Vingegaard. Like the majority of the race, little separated them after the brutal 7km finishing climb of La Super Planche des Belles Filles that culminated in a 24% gradient and gravel stretch to the line. In 2021, Pogačar enjoyed a similarly celebratory 24 hours, winning Pyrenean stages 17 and 18. This ability to go and go again is an indispensable characteristic of Grand Tour winners and, according to an assistant professor in the Division of Endocrinology, Metabolism and Diabetes at the University of Colorado School of Medicine, is all down to Pogačar's blood.

'At the university, we've developed a platform for what's called "metabolomics". With a few drops of blood, we can analyse between 1000 and 2000 parameters of the body,' explains Dr Iñigo San-Millán, who juggles his clinical academic work with coaching Pogačar for UAE Team Emirates. I'd tapped up the Italian as, ultimately, anything blood related in cycling has a bad name. I knew San-Millán was undertaking ground-breaking, legal blood work with cyclists. It might not transfer directly to my own performance but it would certainly satiate my vicarious interest in pro cycling. And who knows, when I'm winning the Tour de France in 2032, I could reflect on my mighty metabolomic profile as the reason why... Back to San-Millán. 'We can understand how the body functions at a level that we've never seen before. Mitochondrial function, cell oxidation, glycolysis, anaerobic capacity, catabolic capacity... We can identify differences between cyclists and see what makes a truly elite athlete.'

And when it comes to Pogačar, it's his extraordinary ability to clear out lactic acid that's been one of the key discoveries from San-Millán's blood work. 'We had Pogačar and 20 other riders at UAE Team Emirates undertake a 15-minute warm-up at relatively low intensity of 2 watts per kilogram [w/kg] of bodyweight. Intensity cranked up by 0.5w/kg every 10 minutes. Power output, heart rate and lactate were measured [via blood extraction] throughout the test, including at the end when the riders were exhausted.

'We discovered that lactate-clearance capacity of the stronger riders was incredible. Let me explain... When a rider's sprinting or climbing, they generate a huge amount of lactate. We call this "highly glycolytic". The problem is, the more your muscles use glucose, the more lactate is produced because it's a by-product of glucose utilisation.

'This lactate builds up and hydrogen ions associated with lactate increase acidosis of the muscle micro-environment, decreasing contraction capacity [power output]. That's why it's critical to clear that lactate. It's been shown that world-class athletes produce more because they have a higher glycolytic capacity and can also clear it more proficiently. Well, Tadej has one of the greatest glycolytic capacities I've ever seen.'

If you're interested in graphs, tables and spreadsheets, search for San-Millán's paper entitled 'Metabolomics of Endurance Capacity in World Tour Professional Cyclists' in the journal *Frontiers in Physiology*[5]. It's a dense but fascinating read.

San-Millán credits the field of metabolomics – aka the scientific study of chemical processes involving metabolites – as steering training content, race selection and even team strategy. 'You can't see what we see with simple blood tests and analysis, and we're the only WorldTour team doing this. Take the Vuelta a España of 2019. Many thought we were crazy to have a 20-year-old [Pogačar] lead the team in his first three-week stage race. Many said he was there for experience and that after 10 or 12 days he'd go home. But we knew different. We knew from his parameters that he could not only recover quickly between in-stage efforts but between stages too. No one improves during a race of that length but it's about reducing the decrement in performance. And that's what Tadej managed, and why the three stage wins he bagged all came in the second and third weeks.'

Critical to Pogačar's ability to recycle lactic acid for energy is the proficiency of his mitochondria. Mitochondria are organelles that reside in your cells and are the furnaces that burn fuel – be it carbohydrates, fats or, if in a state of starvation, protein – for energy. Riders like the two-time Tour de France winner have huge mitochondrial function and are the organelle gold standard.

Pogačar's magnificent mitochondria are fat, as well as lactate, incinerators with San-Millán revealing that while some riders might be burning 80 per cent carbohydrates and 20 per cent fat at a given intensity of training, the Slovenian is the opposite. That's crucial in endurance sport because it means sparing precious glycogen stores – how the body stores glucose in the muscles, liver and brain – for harder parts of the race like an Alpe d'Huez finish. The world's elite max out at around 500g glycogen. That's around 2000 calories of turbo fuel for harder sections. Even wafer-thin Slovenians like Pogačar, whose body fat nestles around 7 per cent, have an endless supply of fat calories to burn though, so if you can train your mitochondria to tap into fat rather than glycogen at higher intensities of exercise, you'll avoid bonking and be able to sustain high power output. All of this detail from a few drops of blood.

San-Millán and his colleagues have perfected the art of examining blood profiles to manage a rider's training programme, to see for instance if a period of hard intervals is best over longer, low-intensity efforts. Unlike Elizabeth Holmes and her Theranos non-start-up (for those who haven't read the book *Bad Blood*, please do – it's a fascinating tale of fraudulently selling tech that doesn't work) the blood tests work, so much so that San-Millán's colleague, Travis Nemkov, is quoted as predicting that the use of metabolite profiles in blood to monitor fitness and exercise regimes could be the sabermetrics of the 21st-century. Sabermetrics is the analysis of baseball statistics in search of improved team performance and was coined by American baseball writer, historian and statistician Bill Jones in 1971. Jones' imprint on one of America's most popular sports proved so important that in 2006 he was included in the *Time* 100 list as one of the most influential people in the world.

Will Iñigo San-Millán, the Spanish-US émigré, be held in similar regard? For sport, perhaps not; for his medical work, maybe. You see, San-Millán is a sports-obsessed cycling coach who formerly played for Real Madrid's academy for five years before swapping studs for cleats and racing professionally, but it's his broader clinical and research work in cellular metabolism that's attracting widespread interest. While Pogačar and co possess peloton-leading mitochondria, at least 50 per cent of the population of the United States don't. And that's something San-Millán's looking to rectify.

'It's a fact that cardiometabolic disease doesn't exist in the elite-endurance population. That's despite the multi-billion dollar weight-loss industry claiming it's all down to too much sugar. Well, professional riders consume tons of the stuff through energy gels and drinks and they're fine.

'Cardiometabolic diseases, like cardiovascular diseases, type-2 diabetes and even Alzheimer's, which will soon be called type-3 diabetes, show one thing in common: mitochondria dysfunction. They can't burn glucose efficiently, meaning glucose builds up, giving rise to insulin resistance and eventually type-2 diabetes. The same things happen with fat. You can't burn it properly, it builds up, leads to inflammatory responses and ultimately cardiovascular disease, weight gain… Mitochondria dysfunction is a big problem.'

Why elites have such impressive mitochondria is down to exercise. Those 30,000km of cycling each year not only lead to huge wattages, lean muscle mass and an impressive vascular network, but they also provide the stimulus mitochondria need to grow and function properly. Without exercise, mitochondria atrophy.

'We know from research that if well-trained athletes stop and become sedentary for two months, their mitochondria drop by 40 per cent. Imagine if you haven't exercised for 20 years? Throw in over-feeding and your mitochondria are overloaded.'

San-Millán doesn't suggest the pre-diabetic population must slip into X-rated polyester, hop on a saddle and pedal up the Dolomites. Walking is a start as even the lightest activity stimulates mitochondria growth. His work reaches well beyond cycling but he's reverted to the world of cycling to highlight the cause with the recently launched Tadej Pogačar Cancer Foundation. It's positive work. Of course, any performance work that involves blood plus links with a cancer foundation echo of times gone by…

While San-Millán is a flag-bearer for the progressive, legal road professional, suggesting that cycling is 100 per cent clean would be naive at best, blinkered at worst. And there are ample examples of suspicious behaviour. For instance, for the second successive year, police stormed the hotel of Bahrain Victorious riders and staff at the 2022 Tour de France. After the raids, Vladimir Miholjević, the Bahrain Victorious performance manager, said that his team was 'sleeping like babies and working like horses'. 'We'd like to know why they are doing this,' Miholjević said of the spate of police searches. At time of print, no one publicly knew and no charges had been made. However, a UCI webinar in May 2022 suggested it was anti-doping's increased focus on intelligence that was behind the suspicion.

'We can't comment on the Bahrain case … but we know from cases like Operación Puerto that testing alone is insufficient,' explained Amina Lanaya, director general at the UCI. 'We know that intelligence and investigation [I&I] is one of our biggest weapons against doping. Cycling can't work alone to break this omerta.' Nicholas Raudenski, who heads up I&I at the International Testing Agency, an independent anti-doping body, added, 'We're going out there and being proactive, digging for information, gathering intelligence. Investigative journalists can appreciate this.'

Repeated knocking on the Bahrain door suggests intelligence is at work. But such open displays of potential improprieties are far rarer than they were in years gone by. The last relatively big scandal to wrap its tentacles around cycling was Operation Aderlass, an investigation in Austria and Germany into doping practices carried out by Erfurt-based German physician Mark Schmidt. It led to the online haranguing of Austrian skier Max Hauke, photographed with a blood bag connected to his arm at the cross-country skiing world championships in Seefeld. Alessandro Petacchi was the highest-profile cyclist to be implicated, the UCI giving the Italian sprinter a two-year ban from competition in 2019, albeit four years after he had retired. But compared to the 1990s, when Lance Armstrong and the Festina Affair dominated the headlines, cycling in the 2020s seems almost puritanical. In fact, in 2020, professional cycling had 'only' the eighth-most doping cases out of 37 sports that registered positive tests according to the Movement for Credible Cycling's 'credibility barometer', dropping three places from the previous year. There were just 18 recorded doping cases compared to 113 in track and field, which held the dubious honour of topping the list. Covid helped massage the figures, of course, but that applied to all sports. Cycling has, surprisingly perhaps, never been top. In 2019, it was fifth – the highest it's been since the MPCC began charting sporting cases in 2014.

While hearsay and gossip will forever hang over professional cycling like a perma-grey cloud, we must take that as good news and there's certainly a feeling that in the 2020s doping practices are the domain of lone wolves rather than the whole pack. 'It seems that the age of strategic team cheating is possibly behind us,' says emeritus professor of biochemistry at the University of Essex, England, and expert in sports doping and biology Chris Cooper. Cooper wrote the book *Run, Swim, Throw, Cheat: The Science Behind Drugs in Sport*[6] and is currently developing an artificial blood substitute. 'Teams continue to stretch the rules on therapeutic use exemptions [TUEs], though.'

TUEs are granted by the World Anti-Doping Agency (WADA) to athletes who have a medical need to take a drug on their prohibited list and came to the fore with the UK Anti-Doping (UKAD) investigation into Team Sky and the notorious 'jiffy bag' incident. Though the Digital, Culture, Media and Sport (DCMS) select committee concluded in 2018 that they weren't in a position to state what was in the jiffy bag delivered to Bradley Wiggins at the 2011 Critérium du Dauphiné, they slated the British team for crossing the ethical line. 'Drugs were being used by Team Sky, within WADA rules, to enhance the performance of riders and not just to treat medical need,' the DCMS report[7] stated. Wiggins was also granted TUEs to take corticosteroids, which can treat allergies and respiratory issues, shortly before the 2011 Tour de France, his 2012 win and the 2013 Giro d'Italia.

While the majority of the team rode off with their careers, if not their reputations, intact, Dr Richard Freeman, one of Team Sky's doctors at the time, admitted 18 of 22 charges against him, such as purchasing the banned Testogel as well as lying to the UKAD. He was permanently struck off the medical register. He appealed but adjournment after adjournment means the case continues. Arguably the bigger issue with TUEs is a welfare one. If a rider's seeking a medical certificate, it's clearly questionable whether they're in a fit state to race.

Core to this cleansing has been the Athlete Biological Passport. Cycling was the first to introduce it in 2008. 'To fiddle the passport is tricky and I feel is the biggest reason why the extreme doping periods of the '90s have dropped,' says Cooper. 'It's not perfect, of course, but it's certainly helped.' Whereas the previous system focused on banned substances – the level and type of erythropoietin (EPO, a hormone that stimulates red blood cell production) in urine, for instance – the passport focuses on anomalous fluctuations in indirect markers of drug abuse over time, the idea being that trends would increase the likelihood of catching cheats.

The WADA-funded passport monitors numerous urine and blood biological variables, including reticulocyte and haemoglobin levels.

A reticulocyte is a new red blood cell. Injecting EPO stimulates the body to produce more reticulocytes, increasing their total percentage. The other primary method of doping, blood transfusion, requires removal of blood before re-infusion. That initial drop screams at the body to compensate by making more red blood cells, again leading to a higher-than-normal percentage of reticulocytes.

This is where things become complicated and where the passport comes in. 'While reticulocytes skew upwards after doping, when you re-infuse your blood [with the blood you stored in the fridge], your actual percentage of reticulocytes then drops because the "older" blood effectively dilutes the new blood,' says Cooper. 'So, the passport picks up if there's unusually high and low reticulocyte levels.'

Haemoglobin plummets when you first extract blood but increases on re-infusion. Comparing the ratio of haemoglobin to reticulocytes gives something called the OFF-score, which picks up both the withdrawal of blood, as well as its re-infusion.

Haematological scientists have observed that most people have reticulocyte percentages between 0.5 and 1.5 per cent. Some are naturally higher or lower but it's the spikes or drops that the testers are eyeing. Though not 100 per cent foolproof, it's created a more stringent system. 'In the past, it was far too easy to mask abuse,' says Cooper. 'I'd say it's much more difficult now.

'The main problem's possibly micro-dosing EPO,' Cooper continues. 'But obviously the smaller amount means less of a performance benefit, so is it worth the risk?'

Maybe, according to convicted ex-rider Joe Papp. Papp's Twitter bio reads: 'Naturalist, Sworn peace officer, Anti-doping advocate, All is ephemeral – fame and the famous as well.' His pinned Tweet is of two images: a smiling Joe with a camera and tripod over his right shoulder on the left; a snowy owl to the right. When we catch up over the phone, he's just been to hospital with his 80-year-old mum; after our call, he'll head over to his brother's house to walk their Labrador puppy. His opening gambit's an update on what he's up to now. 'I'm about to start training to become a law enforcement officer in the state of Pennsylvania ... Only in America could someone with my record climb his way back up to a position of authority and legal responsibility. Pay one's debt to society and become a productive member of it.'

Papp is a former professional cyclist convicted of doping. In 2006, he tested positive for testosterone at the Tour of Turkey and was banned for two years. Just as he was free to start racing again, Papp was charged with drug trafficking, specifically human growth hormone and EPO. According to the attorney, Papp brokered deals worth $80,000 to 187 clients, including cyclists, runners and triathletes. He served a six-month period of house arrest followed by two and a half years' probation, that leniency being down to Papp testifying at the Lance Armstrong and Floyd Landis cases.

Picking up on Copper's comments, Papp believes that micro-dosing EPO could still deliver a 2 per cent performance improvement. In the world of marginal gains, that remains the difference between victory and defeat, of wearing *le maillot jaune* or being swept up by the broom wagon. Micro-dosing's hard to detect because it only skews blood values for a short period. Altitude training can also muddy the waters. Of course, that's nothing compared to the macro-dosing of Papp's days, the time before the passport was introduced.

'I saw a 10–12 per cent improvement in aerobic capacity,' Papp says. 'It gave you wings. I remember a British teammate of mine, Dan Staite, moved to the US to work. We raced a local event together and it was shortly after I started my doping programme in 2001. We broke off the front and I pulled the two of us for nearly two hours. I could inhale all the air in the world to fill my lungs and just ride and ride. He was a better rider than me but clean and hanging off the back. It was amazing the impact it had.' Whether Papp revealed his dark secret to Staite remains to be seen but the British rider tested positive for EPO in 2010.

Papp is a reformed character and open to sharing his litany of prescriptions and doses, including the first EPO prescription he received from a doctor. The handwritten prescription is for EPO drug Procrit, 4000u/ml, single-use vial, six vials, to inject three per week.

He also emailed over the spreadsheet he maintained of the supplementary practices – some legal, many illegal – he employed. It's nine pages long and incredibly detailed. As a snapshot, 'Betamethasone [steroid], 2ml, Jose says it doesn't mark in the controls like those used in Chile so you can take it every day.' 'Diazepam, one tablet per hour before sleeping. Jose recommends this for calming down to sleep after a hard race.' 'Salbutamol, therapeutic dose for adults is 2–4mg administered three or four times a day.' And on it goes. Uppers, downers, it's a Who's Who of the performance-enhancing world.

Despite nearly dying when his haematocrit levels tipped over 60 per cent, Papp's encyclopaedic knowledge of doping products and entrepreneurial skills saw him enter the profitable world of drug trafficking. 'When I was dealing, it was around $50 for a month's worth of EPO and I would sell it for around $500–600,' he explains, before revealing that WADA might be looking in the wrong place. The bigger problem could be something highlighted in the 2015 Cycling Independent Reform Commission (CIRC) report into the state of cycling. 'I'd say about 80 per cent of my clients were recreational riders,' Papp reveals. 'It's why I charged so much. These were type-A personalities who had money to burn. They're highly motivated, mainly men and go all in.' As Cooper suggests, they're also not restricted by the biological passport, which only applies to professionals (though winners of larger amateur events, like L'Étape du Tour, do have to have urine tests). 'I'm sure some amateurs will see it as free rein to dope.'

The pandemic interrupted races – as well as testing – but before the pandemic struck there was a string of doping cases in the recreational ranks. In 2019, two Spanish cyclists were suspended after testing positive for EPO. Forty-five-year-old Raul Portillo won the 45–49 age-group category at the 2018 UCI Gran Fondo World Championships in Varese, with the other rider named as 36-year-old Basque José Antonio Larrea. Closer to home, amateurs Robin Townsend, Andrew Hastings and Jason White all failed doping tests, fitting the identikit profile in the CIRC report of 'middle-aged businessmen winning on illegal products with some of them training as hard as professional riders'.

National 12-hour time trial champion Townsend's case was particularly absurd. He tested positive for the stimulant modafinil, following an in-competition test after finishing ninth at the Burton and District Cycling Alliance 100-mile event in September 2015. Townsend blamed a bitter rival for spiking his drink, the spiker allegedly sending Townsend's partner, Denise Bayliss, a text message 12 months earlier that read: 'You ignorant bastard. That little c*** is only 2 minutes behind me now. I'm going to tear you and him apart.' Though UKAD didn't question Townsend's turbulent relationship with his rival, they did doubt his spiking story.

Doping, it seems, has no age limit. In 2019, Carl Grove set a new record in winning the 90–94 age-group sprint title at the USA Masters Track National Championships, only to test positive for epitrenbolone, a metabolite of trenbolone, which is banned by the United States Anti-Doping Agency (USADA). Grove was stripped of his record and given a public warning but was allowed to race after USADA accepted it was probably caused by consuming contaminated meat the night before the event.

As a recreational rider of no repute, I question why amateurs would cheat. If a professional crosses the line, it's to be rightly condemned, but with mortgages to pay, mouths to feed and anxieties about vocations beyond cycling, the reasons behind it are perhaps understandable, especially in the 1990s when doping was so prevalent. Cheat or retire, those were the choices for some pros. But no-pros drinking, pill-popping and even injecting illegal substances when there is nothing on the line? Just why?

'An academic friend of mine, Michael Shermer, has a fascinating insight into this,' explained Papp. 'He says that ego and pride is [*sic*] just as strong a motivator as money. Men especially are motivated by status and honour in their tribes, going back to our Palaeolithic ancestors. Even just being top dog in a local cycling club can be a real ego boost to a lot of guys, even middle-aged dudes wanting to feel good about their waning powers in search of recapturing their youth.'

Then there's the issue of legal gateway drugs, namely sports supplements. A 2022 study[8] by a team from Canterbury University and Birmingham University, both in the UK, investigated the potential link between moral values, sports supplements and doping.

Morals and values is a key tenet of WADA's strategy, which is 'founded on the intrinsic value of sport'. WADA refers to this intrinsic value as the 'spirit of sport', which is a cornerstone of their doping policy. WADA identifies 11 values that underpin the spirit of the sport, four of which can be classified as moral values: ethics, fair play and honesty; character and education; respect for rules and laws; and respect for self and other competitors.

Five hundred and 60 competitive athletes completed sports-supplement, moral-value and doping questionnaires. For the former, subjects were presented with six statements – for example, 'sports supplements [like caffeine] are necessary for me to be competitive' – and indicated their degree of agreement on a six-point scale, from one (strongly disagree) to six (strongly agree).

The UK team measured one's moral compass using the rather romantic Spirit of Sport Values scale, which asked them to rate the importance of factors like ethics and fair play on a seven-point scale. Doping use was measured using a scale from WADA's Research Package for Anti-Doping Organizations. Athletes were asked to indicate which of the following statements best represents them, from '1) I have never considered using a banned performance enhancing substance' to '7) I regularly try or use banned performance enhancing substances'. For this study, doping use refers to reported doping use.

In both studies, the authors found that sports-supplement beliefs mediated the relationship between sports-supplement use and doping use, and that this mediation didn't exist when moral values and moral identity were high. 'This study is a first at providing evidence that personal morality may influence the relationship between sports supplement use, beliefs and doping, and highlights the important role personal morality plays in an athlete's decision to use prohibited substances.'

With sports-supplement use popular at all levels, the study continued, education is integral to cutting off this pathway, with one study cross-referenced by the UK team reporting 'that young athletes were less likely to dope three and six months after attending a "moral" intervention where participants engaged with content related to the importance of being hardworking, honest and fair'. Whether this preventative measure will work with a 45-year-old banker who should know better remains to be seen. Why? Beyond their middle-aged belligerence, drug testing – especially out of competition – is rare at recreational level. It's hard to say how rare as a body like UKAD, which undertook 2076 tests across numerous sports in the first quarter of 2022, doesn't break down its testing figures into professional and amateur categories. But the elite-only biological blood passport, plus the money swilling around elite sport and wall-to-wall media coverage, suggests it's the world-class sports folk who are under the microscope, not your amateur club mate.

Then again, a friend of mine, Martyn Brunt, does recall one time when doping control's chaperones got their hands on this recreational time-triallist. 'It was the 25-mile National Championships at Etwall,' Brunty regales. 'I was 50 seconds slower than my best so didn't challenge for honours. I was wheeling my bike forlornly back to the car park when I was accosted by a gentleman who told me I'd been randomly selected to be tested.

'I remember having to provide ID, the man explaining that he had to keep me in view the whole time. He seemed quite apologetic but I was OK with it all – it was the only time all day I felt like a proper cyclist! I had to choose two sealed bottles and then went into a cubicle to urinate into one of them – under observation. He watched closely enough to make sure I wasn't filling it from some kind of hidden bladder, I guess. Afterwards I had to tip some into a second bottle, then both were sealed and details written on them, after which I signed a consent form. I was asked if I had taken any kind of medication in the week before the race, which was the only time I became nervous, not because I had but because I couldn't remember if paracetamol counted as a prohibited substance! I was told the sample would be sent off to be tested and I presume nothing untoward was found because I didn't hear anything back.'

Brunty was innocent. As we can see, some aren't. Ultimately, failproof preventative measures are impossible as cheating's clearly a very human trait that transcends far beyond cycling.

'The past few years I've really got into twitching,' said Papp. 'Well, there was an informal year-long county competition here for who could spot the most species of bird. I ended up legitimately becoming the number-one guy in 2020, but I was nearly beaten by a chap who'd won a couple times before it transpired [that he] was submitting fake sightings. I remember seeing a rare bird. Once I reported it, he claimed that he'd seen it, too, at exactly the same spot and exactly the same time. But he wasn't there! Humans are humans. None of us are angels.'

With that, Papp flagged up that it was time to walk his brother's dog, but not before a swan song that pinpointed a further reason why middle-aged men are seen as such easy targets when it comes to doping. 'I received a letter on Friday, which made me laugh. It was from one of the biggest hospital chains in Pittsburgh and had a picture of a baseball player in the corner with the headline quote, "Off your game, Joseph?" It was a pitch for anti-ageing medicine aimed at men with low testosterone levels. This is legit stuff, not some weird Russian pharmacy.' I'm heading towards 46 years old. I feel off my game. Do I have low testosterone level? Am I Joseph? Would I dope in the name of conquering the Étape? Hmmm…

OK, let's switch the browser to the private settings and search 'buy EPO'. Well, would you believe it – at the top of the Google rankings is Russian Pharmacy.net. Papp really knows his stuff. I click on said site to see if I'd lose myself in a moral labyrinth or stay legally on course to conquer/complete my goal event of the Étape.

'Buy EPO online' flashes up with a summer promotion special of two packs of six pre-filled syringes for $295. You can also buy a second pack of Binocrit 2000IU with a 50 per cent discount. This is Amazon on steroids and so blatant. Christ knows what you'd find on the dark web. To be fair to the founders of Russian Pharmacy.net – I couldn't ascertain who they were but the email contact was a chap called Mikhail – they'd done their homework as the detail regarding the physiological role of EPO, its history and its preparation was impressive.

The section on masking agents was particularly illuminating. Papp had mentioned he'd often used aspirin as a blood-thinner. Mikhail and his comrades take it a pharmaceutical step further, explaining that, 'Usually, erythropoietin is found in urine or blood samples. Blood is more likely to be detected than urine. The half-life is five to nine hours, i.e. the detection decreases significantly after two to three days. Heparin [medicine to prevent blood-clotting] is used as a masking agent. Protease injection into the bladder through a catheter is also used.'

Proteases are enzymes that break down proteins. This, according to a 2007 study in the *International Journal of Sports Medicine*[9], is a common technique to 'impede the detection of drugs such as EPO or other peptide hormones'. The extent of the problem is highlighted by the study's prosaic title: 'Proteases in doping control'.

The bladder element is reminiscent of Belgian rider Michel Pollentier, who won the Alpe d'Huez stage to claim the yellow jersey at the 1978 Tour de France. His joy was short-lived, however, as he was caught trying to cheat doping control by holding a pear-shaped tube (condom) beneath his armpit that contained someone else's wee and was connected to his nether regions by a plastic tube. He was subsequently thrown out of the race.

The thought of either injecting my bladder or replicating my bladder via a Durex is enough to banish any thoughts of ignoring the council-tax reminder in favour of blowing the cash on a month's worth of EPO, human growth hormone or the weight-loss drug Xenical. And despite Papp's 10–12 per cent assertions, that would still leave me trailing at the workhorse base rather than the thoroughbred tip of the peloton. Morally, it's probably a touch naughty, too, so instead I opt for a still cutting-edge but legal method of understanding my blood and its impact on performance via a CGM. Diabetics will be well aware of this acronym, standing as it does for continuous glucose monitor. A sensor nestled just beneath the skin measures glucose levels 24 hours a day, seven days a week, transmitting results to an app to help diabetics monitor and track their blood glucose levels and avoid hyperglycaemic or hypoglycaemic episodes.

CGMs are now available to cyclists in the form of Supersapiens, powered by Abbott Libre, the pharmaceutical company that founded the sensor for diabetics. The idea is that non-diabetic cyclists can monitor their blood glucose levels to better plan their nutritional strategies and avoid the dreaded bonk. Bonk, hitting the wall, it's all the same – it's when your body's glucose stores are near empty and suddenly, and rather dramatically, you've gone from managing the sweet spot between effort and speed to riding through treacle. I've been in this sticky situation countless times and discovered ginger cake's the perfect antidote.

The gap Supersapiens spotted derived from modern-day cycling where data is king. Power meters measure your output, heart rate monitors measure how hard you're working but, when it comes to nutrition, old-school trial and error rules.

'And that's where I feel Supersapiens fits in,' Asker Jeukendrup tells me over Zoom. Jeukendrup is a sports-nutrition demigod who works with Jumbo–Visma, home to 2022 Tour de France champion Jonas Vingegaard. He's also a scientific advisor to Supersapiens, alongside sports advisors Chris Froome and Sir Dave Brailsford. 'Power meters and heart rate monitors took a while to catch on, to maximise their use, but now they're mainstays,' the Dutch scientist continues. 'Supersapiens could be the same.'

Not if the UCI has their way. Soon after Supersapiens hit the market, cycling's notoriously conservative governing body banned in-competition use of devices that capture information in metabolic values. EF Education's CEO Jonathan Vaughters took to Twitter to denounce the decision: 'On brand. If they can't understand it, they ban it.' Then again, a product like that from Supersapiens does seem at odds with the UCI's no-needle policy, albeit this applies to 'artificially improving performance or recovery' like injecting vitamins or antioxidants. In the case of Supersapiens, it doesn't directly impact your body in search of stronger riding, just delivers information to do so.

That hasn't stopped the likes of Jumbo–Visma and Jeukendrup using the sensor in training 'with some pretty interesting results'. What those results are, Jeukendrup doesn't disclose, which is either intellectual property or the lure of marketing. Either way, Jeukendrup's sugary flirtation doesn't quell my needle-related trepidation of becoming a Supersapien for a month.

The kit arrives. The key component is an applicator akin to an inflated passport stamp that you press against the upper arm, depositing an ultra-thin filament that's stuck into place by an adhesive sticker. This measures glucose levels in the interstitial fluid (fluid in the body's cells). Puncturing myself with a sensor in the name of performance isn't an easy thought, but one that's much worse than the procedure itself. A sensation similar to the near-imperceptible Pfizer jab is over in a millisecond and there's not even a dull ache.

I've been officially biohacked and will remain that way for the test period. Each biosensor lasts for 14 days and nights and I have two of them. They're not cheap – $150 each – which isn't surprising as the team have racked up millions in investment, presumably from middle-aged businessfolk seduced by the idea of ticking the final empirical box. Happily for my wallet, for the purposes of book research, they sent me a sample.

Still, what price an insight into how I react to a pasty? Will my sugar levels go through the roof if I start the day with Rice Krispies over porridge? Will my glucose become destabilised when riding fasted? And what happens if I choose IPA over H_2O? (I soon discovered that a weekend at an ale festival sends results through the roof, as did drinking Robinsons' finest squash.)

Many questions with unclear answers. On the upside, the sensor proved more comfortable than I'd anticipated, especially in bed, where tossing and turning didn't dislodge the sensor. It slipped beneath my cycle jersey fine and, praise be – stayed put in the rough, tumble and underwhelming quality of Monday-night football.

In fact, through March, when I became a Supersapien, I couldn't believe how imperceptible it was. This was a month when I'd increasingly migrated outdoors for training thanks to my new Vitus road bike. It was cold, meaning layers galore. Base layer, mid-layer and windproof jacket – they all slipped effortlessly over the sensor. I'd also dressed for every outdoor ride in bib longs, two pairs of socks, booties, a Buff and double gloves.

Crisp mornings devoid of clouds were a joy; cool mornings with a grey ceiling above and rain were certainly not. Like my sugar levels, it was an up-and-down month. I'd hit a rhythm of either waking up and heading out for a longer endurance ride – I was intent on becoming a fat-burning machine, both for L'Étape du Tour and for pure, total, ego-driven aesthetics – or waking up and hopping on the Wattbike for efforts that were at a higher intensity than the long, slow aerobic rides but that lasted less than an hour. I'd taken to these shorter-duration, harder efforts instantly as the workload resembled that of my normal run sessions (before I'd gone all TrainingPeaks and focused on two wheels).

Overall, the bike was becoming a good friend, albeit some sessions were certainly more laboured than others. I pointed the finger of blame firmly at that old devil called 'stress'. We'd accepted an offer on our house but were nowhere near finding a replacement. I'd always thought folk were rather hyperbolic when suggesting selling your abode was one of the most chafing jobs you'll undertake. As we scrolled through Rightmove on a daily basis and came up against a barrage of overpriced, undesirable houses, I was now a scrunched-up convert. My rides couldn't help me to entirely escape this irritation. While you might 'feel' fatigue in the legs, it's the brain that's more of a guide. If it's vibrant, pedal away you energised soul. If it's enduring a stress-related blockade, it sucks energy from your limbs like a lethargy-loaded leach.

Anyway, let's return to Supersapiens. Where was I? Ahh, that's it: comfort. It was surprisingly comfortable. But there was a downside, as interpreting the results and then acting on them is a hurdle that may trip up many a rider. Thankfully, I was lucky enough to have Asker Jeukendrup to help. 'Here's an example of how you can use it … If you know your glucose levels are high when you're about to ride, you're very likely to suffer from a rebound hyperglycaemia. If insulin spikes at the same time that your muscle looks to take up glucose, your liver just cannot keep up. As a result, your glucose just drops. So, the advice for the rider is to ensure glucose levels are stable when you start riding.

'I've got a really nice example from Yvonne McGregor,' continued Jeukendrup. McGregor's a legend of the track, who held the British women's hour record until Dame Sarah Storey broke it in 2015. She was born in 1961, still rides hard and, as a marketing tool, is the perfect exemplar of teaching an old dog new tricks.

'McGregor described herself as having a diesel engine. During the first half hour of training, she'd always feel terrible. With the sensor, she discovered that in the first half hour of riding, her glucose dropped. Like every time. And that's partly because she'd eat the same thing for breakfast, wait an hour and then ride. But by doing that, she started her exercise when insulin and glucose were at the peak, leading to a big drop in glucose. And that's why she didn't feel good in the first part of her training ride. So, we experimented with having breakfast half an hour earlier and the composition of that breakfast and she felt a million times better.'

Another person to whom I spoke is Phil Southerland, who's a diabetic himself and founder of Team Type One, an organisation comprised of over 170 athletes with type-1 diabetes, and Novo Nordisk, the UCI ProContinental team. Southerland has used CGM for years and is a keen cyclist. The team and condition inspired the idea of Supersapiens.

'Spend your first week living your life the way you would normally,' Southerland told me. 'If you eat porridge, what happens? If you eat nuts, what happens? At the end of week one, look back at your glucose average. If it's 110mg/dL and you're looking to cut weight, set your target to 100mg/dL. Once you set your exposure, you can plan more efficiently, both over time and in the short term.

'Take power-to-weight ratio. You're looking into what to have for dinner. You look at the app and it shows you're under-exposed to glucose that day. You're not looking to lose weight at the moment so you can have that pizza you were planning. Then again, you look and you're over-exposed to glucose. You've had too much throughout the day, so you know it's salad time with a protein hit like lean chicken. You might go to bed a little hungry but that's fine because you've reached your exposure for the day.'

In theory it's sound and I can see the appeal. The sensors delivered reams of information, such as the fact that for me, butter-coated bagels (I've never been a fan of toppings. Butter, please, and do not tamper) deliver a gentle, stable rise, before dropping slowly. When it came to riding itself, a long effort over two hours – by now, I had two such long-ride staples: Bristol to Clevedon and Bristol to Cheddar Gorge – showed that my glucose levels slowly decreased before rebounding when I consumed an energy gel before this sugary benchmark lowered over time. Intuitive, yes, but visible insight into what's happening below is somewhat empowering, even for a recreational cyclist like myself.

You can then file rides under the 'events' tab for further scrutiny: is sucrose enough or should I add fructose? How many gels should I consume each hour? Why did I bonk? Where did I go wrong?

The CGM is potentially a game changer but not infallible. Critics argue that because glucose is so tightly regulated in non-diabetics, your natural state will level out scores, meaning it's hard to interpret any potential changes. There's also the mix that it's taking its measurements from, which isn't actually blood at all but interstitial fluid. This is the fluid found in spaces around the cells and comes from substances that leak out of blood capillaries. Again, critics argue this leads to inaccuracies.

'Blood is really what we're really interested in, but interstitial fluid will give you the same information,' says Jeukendrup. 'Yes, in certain exercise situations, maybe it's a little bit slow to respond but for the vast majority of cases that doesn't really matter. Generally, we're more interested in periods and … [all we really want to know is] is our glucose stable … before we get on the bike?'

Which arguably suggests that Supersapiens comes into its own more off the bike than on it. Either way, it's an interesting device to play around with and, though expensive, Jeukendrup says you don't need to use it all of the time. Perhaps you could use it as you would a fitness test, taken every couple of months, to reflect and perfect. For me, my ability and my cycling ambitions, having a metal filament inserted beneath the skin feels a little too much. But many could benefit, though there's definitely a learning curve when it comes to interpreting and usefully applying the information.

I'm just about to wave Jeukendrup off our Zoom call, but then I spot a framed Barcelona top in the background. It says Messi and is signed. 'You have a top from the god,' I ask? 'Yes, that's from Lionel, from 2013, I think. I used to work with them [Barcelona FC]. It's one of my most prized possessions. My claim to fame is I've actually shaved his legs. Few people can say that! It was for sweat testing; I put sweat patches on his leg. I had to be careful as I'm sure his legs are insured!' (They are, with his left leg alone reportedly insured for $900 million.)

Supersapiens offered an insight but focused on a very tight remit of glucose metabolism. However, while I was focusing on what lies within, I'd come across Forth Edge, a blood-testing outfit who'd deliver a cycling-specific biomarker profiling service for £99. This piqued my interest since I'd just been talking to coach Phil Mosley, who had supplied me with my training plan, and who had informed me that one in five people in the UK are anaemic or borderline anaemic at any time.

'If I was going on a long drive, I'd want to know before I get in the car whether it'll make the destination, so I'd check in for a service, an MOT,' he said. 'So have a blood test. The GP will do it if you ask nicely. Iron stores, ferritin, B12, vitamin D, magnesium, thyroid activity … all the markers of endurance. They're quite easy to tweak with dietary changes or a supplement. If you're low on iron, for example, it'll feel like a slog. But take an iron supplement, hold on to more oxygen and you feel better.'

It made sense and was certainly cheaper than Supersapiens (although in my case, I'd been lucky enough to once again sidestep that fiscal outlay by waving the media product-testing banner). So,

I ordered a gratis pack, which arrived within a couple of days. The box came with four lancets, two microcontainers, alcohol-cleansing wipes and detailed instructions. I had to warm up my hands and then prick my finger, squeeze and drop blood into the containers. I've given blood for years so I'm used to a temporary puncture to top up stocks. (Unlike the Supersapiens, which threw me at the start because of both the 24-hour insert and the fact it was for sporting, not medical, reasons.) But you must be precise. Hit the right spot on the fingertip (the side of your ring or third fingertip) and the red stuff flows. Fail to and you'll barely find a droplet, meaning you'll need lance after lance. I managed the procedure, cleaned up the puncture wound, packed up the self-addressed box and sent it to the lab. Within a few days, the results arrived via the app.

The results? Well, all reassuringly fine as I sat in the middle of 'normal' in most categories. How reliable were the results? The sceptic in me contacted Forth Edge to ensure all was medically sound. Fair play, they replied quick-smart. 'The normal reference range in the majority of cases is set by the assay manufacturer and is based on the research they have undertaken for their particular product. The "normal" range is calculated as the range in which 95 per cent of a healthy population falls into. On some markers such as vitamin D or cholesterol, ranges are set by health governing bodies.' They also confirmed they only use laboratories with something called UKAS accreditation ISO 15189. 'It's the gold standard in the industry and the same standard met by NHS laboratories,' they concluded. I'm convinced – the results are valid. And here they are…

- Vitamin B12. Absorbed via diet and plays a role in the production of red blood cells and in nerve health (it helps to maintain the sheath around nerve cells called myelin). It's an essential vitamin as you can't make it yourself. Lack of it leads to anaemia. It can only be derived in the diet from animal sources such as meat, fish and dairy, so is often deficient in vegetarians, so they need to take a supplement.

My score: 92.8 picomoles per litre [pmol/L] (normal). Forth average 118.84 pmol/L.

- Cortisol. A steroid hormone released when the body's under stress. Anxiety, a restricted diet or overtraining can cause a rise. If it's too high or low, you feel weak.

My score: 309 nanomoles per litre [nmol/L] (normal). Forth average 367.46 nmol/L.

- Vitamin D. Plays an essential role in healthy bones, immune system and muscle function, to name but three.

My score: 88.4 nmol/L (normal). No Forth average figure given.

- Ferritin. Reflects the total level of iron stored in the body. Can be raised due to inflammation. The best source is red meat.

My score: 81.8 micrograms per litre [ug/L] (just in normal range). Forth average: 204.66 ug/L.

- Testosterone. A hormone that plays an important role throughout the body, including in maintaining muscle mass. Naturally declines with age. Strength work helps raise levels.

My score: 16.8 nmol/L (normal). Forth average: 18.6 nmol/L.

And on it went. It was appreciatingly detailed. I was pleased that the vitamin D score looked OK – I'd taken a supplement all winter due to lack of sun. However, my ferritin levels were a little low, which wouldn't be great for the mountains of France.

I was surprised cortisol levels weren't higher; in fact, the only marker that came up high was creatine kinase. This is an enzyme mainly found in the brain, heart and skeletal muscles. It's released into our muscles when they are damaged to create a rapid source of energy that can be used for muscle contraction. However, if muscles become stressed, injured or inflamed, they leak cytosolic enzymes including creatine kinase. My score was 410 units per litre (U/L) compared to the Forth average 196.76 U/L. This added up as I'd had football the evening before and my legs were battered.

My haemoglobin levels were also borderline high. This is the protein found in red blood cells that's responsible for carrying oxygen to other cells in the body. Above-average is a sign of dehydration, and again smacked of me not hydrating well enough post-kickabout.

But in general, the results were promising. As was the training. I'd improved my FTP score to 230 watts, which changed the zones on my TrainingPeaks app, which made me far too delighted. It also made each session harder, which I guess is the payback for progress. We were into spring and L'Étape du Tour on 10 July was edging closer. Life was busy, work was busy, family were very busy/demanding. After the break-in, it had transpired that life wasn't cobbles after all. Or was it…

5

The Lion Meets the Pussy Cat

T-minus three and a half months

The Tour of Flanders, also known as De Ronde, is one of the five Monuments, the events that are deemed the hardest and most prestigious in cycling. Milan–San Remo, Paris Roubaix, Liège–Bastogne–Liège and Giro di Lombardia are the other four, but for Flandriens, there is only one.

'It's all about the cobbles and the hills. Koppenberg is a mythical climb. Paterberg is a mythical climb. Kwaremont is a mythical climb. There are many mythical climbs. It's why Flanders is so famous. It's why Flanders is so spectacular.' These are the words of Johan Museeuw or 'The Lion of Flanders' to Belgians – a man who'll offer unique insight into one of the world's toughest one-day races, which is arguably the biggest cycling race on the spring calendar.

It's April, it's still chilly but the cycling season is hotting up – both for the professionals and this ageing amateur. Like nearly every major professional cycling event, the Tour of Flanders hosts an accompanying recreational ride. These sportives are big business, with events like my goal event, L'Étape du Tour, selling out in hours. As a build-up to my Alpine odyssey, and to experience the unique rough and tumble of the cobbles, I'd decided to shadow the professionals by not just digging deep into their experiences but also enduring those vibrations myself. In short, I'd join 16,000 others at the Tour of Flanders Sportive. It'd be a gauge of the success my training and hopefully deliver a competitive boost of motivation.

And who better to deliver a motivational talk and advice than Museeuw, who raced professionally between 1988 and 2004, winning Paris–Roubaix three times, the world championships in 1996, plus two stages of the Tour de France? That said, it's his three victories at Flanders – a record held with five other men, including fellow Belgians Tom Boonen and Achiel Buysse – that lionised the now 56-year-old.

Museeuw was arguably the greatest classics rider of a generation and, in a sport fuelled by its strongman reputation, 'The Lion' was one of the toughest of them all, thriving on the cobbles that'd leave many licking their wounds. His determination, his capacity to dig deeper than the farmers who plough this land, stemmed from his desire to win. Museeuw didn't *have* to win, he *needed* to win. It's a competitive instinct that burns bright to this day.

'I might have won three times but I also finished second three times and third three times,' he tells me over the phone in a softly spoken voice at odds with his muscle-man image. 'For some riders, that's OK. For the sponsors, hitting the podium is OK. It wasn't for me. There was only one place that counted and that was number one.'

In 1998, Museeuw suffered a horrendous crash at Paris–Roubaix that left him with a shattered kneecap. Infection set in and doctors considered amputation. A year later, he was riding to one of those third-place finishes at Flanders. It left Museeuw with a deep scar and it's still not as profound as defeat.

'Flanders is always hard. But the pain is less when you win. I remember back in 1994, I came second to Gianni Bugno by the smallest distance in the history of the race [quoted as 7mm]. I was in good shape and a good position with 200m to go but made a bad mistake, starting my sprint before Bugno not after him. You don't have two chances in sport and I messed that one up.'

Museeuw lives in Oudenaarde, where the 2022 men's race finished. It started in Antwerp and measured 272.5km. The women's event started and finished in Oudenaarde, and came in at 159.8km long. Museeuw was born and raised here, too, so he is moulded by the land and sweeping downpours common at this time of year.

Growing up, his first sport was football and he rarely touched the bike. But soon cycling and the cobbles took hold and Flanders became his painful, but pleasurable, playground. 'I never really had to do specific course reconnaissance work as I know this region so well. I've ridden the cobblestones, the climbs, the corners from an early age, so when I turned professional I felt confident that I'd do well here. It's our history, our culture. It's in the blood.'

It's that combination of cobblestones and climbs that's chiselled out its brutal reputation. Yes, the total pavé of the 2022 men's race rolled to less than 20km compared to Paris–Roubaix's 50km-plus, but they lay the vibration-inducing, muscle-fatiguing foundations for the majority of the climbs. Roubaix, while more cobbled, is generally flatter.

It's a parcours that would rattle the sub-60kg Tour climbers into submission. This is a race that demands an anatomy loaded with muscle and power, and is why Museeuw asserts that his race weight was always 75kg. 'OK, a couple times it might have been 1kg more, and I'd lose 1kg for the Tour and its bigger mountains, but I was pretty much set at 75kg the entire year. I wasn't one of those riders who'd take five or six weeks off in the winter and pile on 5 or 6kg. I'd have two weeks off and then start training.'

In Museeuw's day, brutality was measured by the blood, sweat and (very rarely) tears dripping down one's face. Nowadays, it's all about the empirical. Mathieu van der Poel uploaded his 2021 Flanders data, where he finished second to Quick-Step's Kasper Asgreen, to Strava, revealing that he averaged 41.9km/h for the six-hours-plus of racing, generated by an average 328 watts, including a huge 1470-watt (yes, really, you read that right!) effort in the final sprint for the line. In the process, the Dutch phenomenon broke numerous King of the Mountains (KoM) records, including the devastating double finale of Oude Kwaremont and Paterberg, treating them like dimples as he stormed the two iconic climbs in 8.50 minutes at an average 420 watts.

That's despite the unique physical challenge of the cobbles. Or, more appropriately, 'specific' challenges of the cobbles as studies into their impact on the body have generally focused on Roubaix rather than Flanders. Take research by sports scientist and amateur rider

Sébastian Duc of Reims University, France, who signed up to the 2015 Paris–Roubaix sportive in an attempt to understand the deleterious effects of the cobbles.

Duc attached a duo of tri-axial accelerometers to his Specialized Roubaix, a bike the American manufacturers designed and created specifically for the demands of the cobbles, clamping one to the stem and one to the seatpost. These micro-devices recorded the vibrations shuddering through Duc and his Roubaix in an effort to isolate where the greatest pain is endured.

'This is important,' the Frenchman told me from his Reims home. 'Vibrations can induce many symptoms and injuries in cyclists, including numbness in the fingers [due to ulnar nerve compression], loss of gripping force, muscle aches and pains in the arms, shoulders, back, a sagging of the skin on the hands and buttocks due to overpressure and repeated shocks. . .'

I'm sure we'd all spend on products that wouldn't leave us with saggy buttocks. I digress. Duc's challenge comprised 139km and 15 cobble segments, ranging from the euphemistic 'easy' (two stars) to 'very hard' (five stars). The lithe Duc hit the scales at 68kg and was 1.80m tall, so arguably designed more for smooth vertiginous roads than jagged lumps of rock.

Nevertheless, Duc negotiated the hazards in style, averaging 28.1km/h at an intensity that saw his heart oscillate between 122 and 155bpm. Cadence flowed from 79 to 89rpm while his power output ranged from 167 to 235 watts. That's the physiological top line but what about the results generated by the tri-axial twins?

'As expected, the ferocity of vibrations measured at the stem [hand] and seatpost [whole body] increased with the cobbles' difficulty,' Duc explained. 'More specifically, what we call the "vibrational value" reached $35m/s^2$ at the stem and $28m/s^2$ at the seatpost.'

As I'm sure you're all fully clued up on, health-and-safety regulations stipulate that anything over $10m/s^2$ is deemed dangerous. We're talking a farmer ploughing a field rather than a keyboard-tapper like me. What does that mean for pavé-heavy races like Flanders and Roubaix, beyond cancellation? Should bike manufacturers and riders focus their damping resolutions at the front end of their bikes? Maybe not, according to Duc. 'The frequency of vibrations was actually higher at the seatpost. As an example, over the three-star sections of cobbles, we measured 30 hertz [Hz] at the seatpost compared to around 20Hz at the stem.' In other words, less intense but more numerous.

Duc suggested that the secret to if not conquering the cobbles but at least reducing their jarring effects is simple: you need to ride fast. 'Also, choose an adequate gear ratio [not too small but not too big]. I think the ideal pedalling frequency is close to 80–85rpm. Basically, if the cyclist moves too slowly, he'll feel all the impact.'

Damn.

In today's peloton, cobble-specific gear is big business. As a snapshot, the Trek Madone SLR7, as used by the Trek–Segafredo men's and women's teams for the pavé, employs what the marketing crew call 'the adjustable top-tube IsoSpeed'. It might not be catchy, but it is rather clever. While retaining the diamond-shaped frame geometry that John Kemp Starley's safety bike featured all the way back in 1885, the seat tube and top tube are 'decoupled', allowing the seat tube to flex with the forces of the turbulent terrain. That cleverness comes at a price, of course, and it's yours for a cobble's width under £9000.

Then there's that Roubaix of Specialized, named after the eponymous bone-shattering Hell of the North. Its USP is the dramatic 'Future Shock'. While their North American rivals focused their efforts out back, Specialized looked up front, slotting in the Future Shock above the head tube to provide up to 20mm travel. Again, you'll need deep pockets to smooth out the deep crevices, the electronic groupset version coming in at over £12,000.

Arguably, these vibration-dampeners are reserved for Roubaix, where the cobbles are deeper and so more jarring. They're notoriously unforgiving but still require a degree of TLC to be kept in good, brutal order. It's why every year Les Amis de Paris–Roubaix, the Friends of Roubaix spend late winter ensuring they're in perfect condition. The 'friends' employ heavy metal farming equipment to ease the cobbles back into the mud, guaranteeing they're rideable but will still leave their imprint in the riders' bones for months to come.

'Thankfully, the cobbles of Flanders aren't as debilitating, albeit they're still tough,' Bob Jungels, the Luxemburg rider, told me in the week leading up to Ronde. Jungels is more at home in the Ardennes classics later in the month, his palmarès including victory at Liège–Bastogne–Liège in 2018. Since then, he's endured a torrid time due to a debilitating condition that was identified in 2021 as arterial endofibrosis, which is essentially restricted blood flow around the hips from scar tissue forming over millions of pedal strokes. Symptoms are fatigue and a loss of power, and it's certainly not ideal when facing the cobbles. Thankfully, surgery's worked and Jungels would later go on to win a stage of the 2022 Tour de France. But back to Jungels' gear thoughts.

'I'll use my standard BMC road bike but will pay great focus to the tyres,' he explained. 'Some might use 30mm-wide tyres but I'll go for 28mm as there are long stretches of road between the cobbles.' Logged. 'I'll pay close attention to clothing, too, as it can be very cold in Flanders at this time of year. It's especially important to retain warmth at the start when you're hanging around, though you'll want your body to breathe later on as you heat up. I'll begin by layering up with leg warmers, gilet and possibly shoe covers. Some guys might even wear a headband or cap plus thick gloves. Once the blood's flowing, I'll remove them and throw them to the soigneurs at the side of the road or to the team car.'

Another note to self: either employ a squad of soigneurs to line the Flandrean roads for heat-regulation purposes or work out what clothes are needed – and, more importantly, how I'll store them if I feel the need to whip them off – for the change in temperature.

I imagine Museeuw, as thickset as the neat, cemented rows of cobbles, would pour scorn on fleece-lined gloves and cranium-cradling caps. And true to form, Getty Image's photo archive is populated by myriad images of a young Museeuw bedecked in a short-sleeved Mapei cycle top and bib shorts, battling the competition against leafless trees and triple-layered spectators. Like Jungels, however, bike gear changes focused on rubber.

'We didn't have 28 or 30mm tyres like they have today,' Museeuw said. 'They're great for rolling over the tougher terrain without compromising speed. We settled for thinner 22mm tyres. We'd deflate the tyre pressure to better cope with the cobbles but only to around 100psi. Any more and the thinness of the wheel could lead to a puncture. Now, with those wider wheels and tyres, you have riders racing at about 70psi. Again, because of the wheel-and-tyre design, they don't lose speed but do retain comfort.'

This penchant for wider tyres is worth a deeper dive. In Museeuw's day, thinner was always thought faster, the logical conclusion that the less the contact with the ground, the less rolling resistance between tyre and ground. Also, a thinner tyre is lighter. Things changed around 2013 when teams like the now-defunct BMC Racing switched to 25mm for traditional road events after research showed that a tyre that width was around 7 per cent faster than a 22mm version. This was down to two key reasons.

The first is that the wider tyre would fit better on to the wheel and so smooth out airflow where the two meet. The second is because of something called tyre deflection. At the same tyre pressure, a wide and narrow tyre has the same contact area as a thinner tyre because while the wide tyre is flattened over its width, the narrower tyre flattens over its length. They're also more comfortable than thinner tyres because of the greater volume of air between the rider and the road. This 'wider is faster and more comfortable' mantra naturally migrated to the cobbles a year later, when teams started using 28mm-thick tyres over more jagged terrain. Now, with the advent of disc-brake bikes, frames can accommodate even wider tyres if the situation demands. Tyres tend to be tubeless these days, too, meaning an inner tube is not required; instead, the tyre is sealed with sealant. The benefits of this are that you can run the tyres at slightly lower air pressure, which maintains good speed but also aids grip and comfort. And if you puncture, the sealant should immediately plaster the hole without you even knowing. Basically, I need width and tubeless.

Despite Starley's triangular geometry surviving the passage of time, bike gearing has evolved beyond recognition since Museeuw's day. Carbon proliferates, gears are shifted wirelessly and electronically, and it's rare a professional or recreational rider's handlebars don't feature a smartphone-sized bike computer containing more technology than CERN. The parties have evolved, too, due to a change in the calendar.

'I never really celebrated my Flanders wins because when I raced, [the classic] Gent–Wevelgem was on the Wednesday after,' Museeuw laments. 'In the evening, we might have a glass or two of champagne but nothing more as the next day you had to recover and train.'

Now, Gent–Wevelgem's the Sunday before and, for many riders, Flanders signals the end of a tough spring calendar. They'll enjoy a rest, race a few week-long stage races, attend altitude camps and then hit the Tour. But they will raise a glass or two after Flanders first.

Which naturally brings up the topic of beer. Flanders has carved a reputation as April's version of Oktoberfest, hundreds of thousands of spectators lining the parcours to cheer on the pros while aiming to remain upright after kick-starting a meticulous all-day Duval-drinking programme while the riders were still to consume their pre-race rice and omelette. Beer and Belgium are synonymous, which begs the question: what does a three-time Flanders hardman drink to lubricate his still granite limbs (he still cycles over 1000km a month; just play voyeur and look him up on Strava)? And, nearly 20 years after he retired, where does he consume said drink when watching the Tour of Flanders?

'I don't have a favourite because I'm not a beer drinker. I know that's very strange for a Belgian to say. I'm actually a red-wine fan from days racing for Mapei [1994–2000]. My favourite is a Sassicaia or a Masseto but they're quite expensive so mostly I'll go for something cheap like a €15 bottle.'

Cheap? That's crossed the double-digit Rubicon de Vin that I promise never to tread.

'As for where I watch, I often decide on the day. Sometimes I might be in an organiser's car. Often not, though, as Flanders week is always busy. Because I still live in Oudenaarde and close to the finish, many times I'll head to Antwerp for the start, go home to watch it on television and then walk over to watch the finish. To be honest, I love to stay home and watch. It's so busy and you're obviously recognised because they are cycling fans.'

And they really are. Think Lionel Messi and the Catalan devotion or Michael Jordan's Chicago love-in. A Belgian winning Flanders means you'll never have to buy another beer, or glass of red wine, again. That adulation can easily seep over into suffocation, of course, and is something fellow three-time winner Tom Boonen told me about in an interview during my last mainland European gig before Covid hit.

'I prefer watching it here on my own,' Boonen confessed when I met him at his Mol home, not too far from Antwerp. 'For two years I went to Flanders, just visiting spots and watching the race from the big VIP area. But everybody's getting drunk and asking me questions, and I just want to watch the race.

'You feel out of place as you want to sit on the bicycle. You have more control of the situation on the bike and in the race. You have a sense of adrenaline to keep you on your toes. But if you're watching it, you have control over nothing.'

That control resonates with Museeuw's previous comments about fearing no one. Like Museeuw, Boonen was good company and, like the early retired Museeuw, enjoyed the fruits of his Flandrean success, his recently renovated Mol farmhouse a permanent reminder of the fiscal benefits. It really was beautiful. And quirky. And a trip down memory lane. Beside a waist-sided rainbow-coloured elephant stood a four-tier shelf, each straining beneath the weight of cobbles collected in 2005, 2008, 2009 and 2012 from his Roubaix victories. Bronze sculptures faced the cobbles, each won at Flanders. They were both dwarfed by a shiny trophy that resembled football's European Champions League cup.

'That's from winning a 24-hour race in Dubai this January,' he revealed. 'I had to dismantle it for customs!' It was the maiden victory for Boonen's Belgian racing team in a series titled 24H Series, during which three drivers rotate. Boonen's cycling success fuelled his latest passion of motorsport and he dreams of racing Le Mans.

If you want to feel very poor and very slow, visit Boonen. In his garage hang the driving overalls of two-time world superbike champion Colin Edwards beside the rainbow jersey he won in 2005, overlooking a Porsche 964 Turbo that Boonen spent years restoring behind a Specialized S-Works with vivid gold decal. Again, funded by his worlds' victory. Reassuringly, and unlike Museeuw, there was also a fridge packed with beer albeit with the words 'No mayo, low salt' scrawled in a heart on the glass door.

Boonen had further Porsches in storage, plus an old Norma he used to drive. And just for good measure, he's even taken to selling cars. 'The showroom's called Iconic Cars,' he explained. 'Essentially, we take overstock from car manufacturers and sell them on. There are some normal cars but a few are really special. We've sold two McLaren P1s, an Aston Martin One-77 and a Bugatti Veyron.'

Before I left, Boonen looked to the future.

'I was there when Mathieu [van der Poel] was trying to come back on the Kwaremont and the speed he passed by was incredible. I don't want to compare myself with Mathieu but if there's one thing I see in both of us, it's how we race. He throws all his cards on the table and isn't afraid to finish second. It's all or nothing and that's more satisfying. Take my last Flanders [2019]. Instead of looking to break on the Kwaremont, like countless editions, we pushed hard on the Muur with about 100km to go. That broke the pack and about 15 of us went clear. People thought we'd never stay away. But it worked as [teammate Philippe] Gilbert won.'

Boonen and Museeuw are legends of the cobbles. When they speak, you listen. What are the main takeaways? From both riders – explicitly in Museeuw's case, just a look of the eyes in Boonen's – a race is always more painful when you don't win. Which explains the deep pain I've endured in all endurance events I've ever completed and the inevitable pain of L'Étape du Tour. On the upside, it's clear that weight (or lack of it) will be more important in the Alpine mountains than upon a cobbled parcours like Flanders. Tyre choice and pressure are more critical on the cobbles than any other terrain. Ultimately, advice only gets you so far. Knowledge is important but you can only truly experience something when you live it…

By the end of Sunday, 3 April 2022, the beer flowed over Mathieu van der Poel and Lotte Kopecky after they both sprinted to Flanders victory.

But that was an afterthought for the event ~~every~~(no)one was talking about 24 hours earlier: the War of Worcester. After three months of TrainingPeaks guided training, I could feel my fitness growing and, despite my 45 creaky years, Phil Burt's positional tweaks had ensured that pains, strains and general disdain were absent. I'd even begun to enjoy the long ride, with Harry Pearson's fantastic account of the spring classics season – *The Beast, the Emperor and the Milkman* (Bloomsbury, 2019) – accompanying each pedal stroke via audiobook. Granted, the weight wasn't dropping off, but I took comfort in Museeuw's and elite coach Dan Healey's words: that it was important to build strength before cutting pounds. I knew the likes of classics riders and sprinter Thor Hushovd would lose several kilograms between the cobbled season and the Tour. That was about three months, which was the same period between me and my Étape du Torture. If that was sufficient for The God of Thunder, it was good enough for this mere mortal.

I'd signed up to the Tour of Flanders sportive – held the day before the pro's event – as part of mimicking the pro calendar for a reasonable €65. Not only would the event be fun (in hindsight, anyway), it'd be a clear indication of whether the training was having the desired impact. I was under no illusions, however – this would be one long, sore day in the saddle. By now, three months into my six-month structured plan, my longest weekly endurance ride was touching three hours. Flanders would be at least double that, upon testicularly terrifying terrain. I'm sure such a skew in my training wouldn't be recommended. Still, I could test out hydration and fuelling strategies. And the pure logistics of getting from A to B and then racing. And anyway, I'd endured this leap into the race unknown many times before. When I had completed the London Marathon, I had barely trained over 18 miles. Of course, I had felt that lack of mileage come the race but, though a broken man and with dribble seeping from most orifices, I had finished in under four hours. Not too bad, I thought, although I was still very much a completer rather than a competer. But I'm happy with that. I don't have enough demons to be the total competitor!

So, Tour of Flanders sportive it would be. This was decided after chatting to the Angelic Cherub and bike mechanic Greg Lancaster back home in Bristol. He'd ridden Flanders and Roubaix and said he'd never ride Roubaix again. Decision made. An easy one. I then put the call out to good friends Timbo and Kempo, aka Tim Jackson and Ian Kemp. (The addition of an 'o' to either a forename or surname is nicknaming of the laziest order and something I inherited from growing up playing football; that said, it's not just me. I'm Jimbo to Timbo.) We met at the University of Worcester, stayed good friends and now all three of us to some degree cycle. 'It'll be easy,' I lied. 'Certainly easier than looking after the kids.' They both have two children under 10 so I thought that bit might be true. They agreed.

Four distances on offer cover the spectrum of abilities and ambition: 75km, 144km, 179km and 235km. All would start and finish in Oudenaarde apart from the 235km option, which would start in Bruges. That was never an option. Timbo's the head-down, emotionally detached type, so would have happily chosen 179km. I had reservations about the cobbles, so pitched for 144km. Kempo's the least experienced, so contemplated the 75km. 'It's a long way to travel [to cycle] for less than 50 miles, Kempo,' Timbo proclaimed with an empathy he's renowned for. We settled on the 144km option.

As this was my gig, it was down to me to look after logistics, starting with our mode of transport to Belgium. Kempo lives in Worcestershire, Timbo in Bromley and I in Bristol – a disparate set-up that didn't lend itself to flying. London has regular flights to Brussels, the nearest airport to Oudenaarde, but that's a bit of a trek from the West, plus you still have 70km to Oudenaarde the other end. Plane ticket prices are good but not with the added bike boxes. And none of us had travelled abroad with a bike box before. We could hire bikes there, but I for one wanted to ride the Vitus I'd come to love, even if it wasn't strictly the perfect road bike for the cobbles. And then there's the environmental cost of flying.

So, Eurotunnel it was, at a very reasonable £135 return. That was £45 each. I'd train it to Kempo's in Worcestershire, he'd drive us to Timbo's in Bromley, we'd stay the night and then drive to Belgium the next morning, our bikes clamped to Timbo's neat Thule roof racks. Entry and travel down, accommodation to go.

Our relatively late race entry meant Oudenaarde was out. Still, Gent's the largest city in east Flanders, only a half-hour drive away, and had options. Kempo, programme officer that he is, couldn't resist a stab at playing Judith Chalmers of *Wish You Were Here* fame but seemed to favour overly priced, sterile, corporate hotels that could have been anywhere. 'I'll source something cheaper and with character,' I assured all.

And I did: the 'Casa Lucinda'. The owners had returned 'Lucinda' to its early 1900s pomp with chandeliers, stove and even four-poster beds. That last addition would arguably be wasted on this trio but the hearty breakfast, billiards table and free beer on arrival would not. OK, it looked a little kitsch on the website, especially the sepia pictures of the owners dressed up in early 1900s Belgian fancy dress, but I was after character and this looked like it had it in bucketloads.

We'd stay three nights – Friday to Monday – and it would cost us £425 in total, so just over £140 each. Not accounting for petrol to fuel movements in England, France and Belgium or motorway tolls, the Eurotunnel fee, race entry and shelter would cost us around £250 each. Yes, that's more expensive than attending a sportive at home but it's not bad for the opportunity to race on the shoulders of giants, and certainly nothing like the extortionate price of racing an Ironman triathlon.

The plan is set. Thursday night and Friday morning travel; Friday afternoon register; Saturday conquer the sportive; Sunday recover with protein shakes, compression socks and an easy ride (alternatively, watch the professional race in heavily drunken fashion alongside the locals –when in Rome…); Monday home.

I arrive at Kempo's off a good block of training both on the turbo and on the road despite a few days off the bike due to late-winter sniffles. In fact, as this represented roughly the midway point to my no-pro journey, it's timely to reflect on how a training week was looking in the life of Tadej Witts, though I'll reel back a couple weeks to mid-March. At this point, I hit a bump in the training road, since I was not only easing off the training slightly in the week before Belgium, but also because I had to take my son on a trip to attend the Newcastle University open day. This involved three days of hotels, university tours and work with no Wattbike or Vitus to hand. The alternative was a very tired hotel gym where the indoor bike creaked and the room reeked.

So, what follows is a snapshot of my training up to mid-March, highlighting how five-a-side football and occasional bike commutes complemented the formalised bike training:

Monday 7 March: 60-minute five-a-side football, plus two 40-minute bike rides to football and back. I'd usually drive to football but my wife had the car. Needless to say, this was rather tiring.

Tuesday 8 March: 20-minute commute to work; electric scooter home.

Wednesday 9 March: a 41-minute M.A.P. effort session on the Wattbike. The purpose of this workout – a common one in my plan – is to not only improve my aerobic capacity, but also to crank up my ability to generate greater power over short intervals, like a short, stiff hill. The warm-up consists of seven minutes on zone two (around 56–75 per cent of my maximum power output), followed by a 10-second burst in zone five (106–120 per cent of my max). This is to prepare for the main set. I do five of these 10-second bursts with 50-second intervals in zone two in-between. Warm-up complete, the main set consists of 90 seconds on zone five with 90-second recoveries in zone two. I do this seven times, usually in an increasingly sweaty state. There's then a five-minute warm-down in zone two.

Thursday 10 March: a day off, which is good as my notes on the TrainingPeaks app read: 'Felt very tired'!

Friday 11 March: a half-hour easy commute.

Saturday 12 March: a 57-minute endurance ride.

Sunday 13 March: a 2.30-hour endurance ride. The rides on Saturday and Sunday crank up the volume, which is needed for events like Flanders and L'Étape du Tour, but as both are relatively low intensity, they can easily follow each other without me ending up in the foetal position on the sofa.

So, training up to Flanders was if not perfect, at least sufficient enough for me to feel in bright nick. But there were clouds. My wife had just contracted Covid; I tested negative. Little did we know that my poor wife would still be struggling with long Covid many months later. And in the week prior to Flanders, I'd felt deep sadness over the death of The Cycling Podcast's Richard Moore, who tragically died in his sleep at the age of just 48. I'd been a fan of Moore, Daniel Friebe and Lionel Birnie for years, and had also met Richard a fair few times at races. He had a warmth, easy charm and humour that touched many, including me. His name will live on through his body of work and I recommend you read his back catalogue, including the excellent *Dirtiest Race in History* about the 1988 Olympic 100m final.

Still, when I arrive at Kempo's house, he's like a loveable puppy and brightens the mood. We drive to Timbo's, kip, wake early, load up the bikes, drink coffee and drive to Folkestone. That's all good. What isn't is the torrential rain sweeping over Kent that soon morphs into a hailstorm and then snow. I'd seen the forecast, packed appropriately (including two pairs of gloves) but seeing is believing. And that seeing is making me believe that if this weather holds just 250km away in 24 hours' time, we're in for a long, saturated, chafing, frozen, distressing day in the saddle.

Which pretty much sums up the life of a lorry driver right then as the queues out of Folkestone stretch back over 32km. Reports of the tailbacks had been on the news but seeing it for yourself evokes a much stronger emotion – especially when those queues threaten our leaving slot, which we'd swiftly calculated could cost us another £300. One of the glories of cycling for all three of us derives from escaping for that one moment in time, of clearing negative thoughts and welcoming positive ones. Now, we're in a stationary metal box enduring the double hit of climate change and Brexit. This isn't the stress-free warm-up we were after. Thankfully, Eurotunnel are surprisingly empathetic, so our later departure comes at no extra expense and we're soon leaving Calais.

The drive through northern France and into Belgium is bleaker than normal. I love both countries. The Vendée, Lyon, Marseillan Plage … stunning, stunning, stunning. The Belgian people? Self-deprecating, funny and generous. But this industrial hinterland in these weather conditions is dire.

I'm hungry, too. We haven't had breakfast and Timbo's keen to sign on at registration in Oudenaarde, so we pass service station after service station. This carbo drought's not ideal with over six hours' riding tomorrow. Thankfully, mood salvation comes in the form of Oudenaarde and a ceasefire in wet hostilities. We park up, sign up, but don't fuel up. There are no feeding options nearby so, starved of choice, en route to 'Lucinda' we stop for a McDonald's. I choose a chicken burger and fries, convincing myself this is protein and carbohydrate of the highest order, and we head off.

'Casa Lucinda' turns out to be even more characterful than I'd thought with a basement that had a haunting feel akin to *Rentaghost*, one of my favourite 1980s' children's programmes. There was definitely no way any of us was going into the cellar. But the rest of the hotel would prove a wonderful place to stay and the hosts, Mindy and her chap, couldn't do enough for us, serving up the most delectable breakfast spread of cheese, tomatoes, hams and pastries – which arguably was the best fuelling we'd enjoy all weekend as our last supper comprised a tuna Domino's pizza. 'It's carb loading,' I tell the chaps.

To be fair, Timbo is too busy for pizza. And too stressed. He's broken rule number one of Sportive Club, which was never, ever attempt to change a bicycle chain the night before the big event. 'Don't do it,' we warn Timbo. 'I do it all the time, changing almost every month.' Blimey, that's keen if not extreme, I thought. Well, good luck to you. The last time I fixed a chain it took repeated orders on Wiggle as I kept ballsing-up the chain masterlink. Like chefs and hospitality staff in general, a good mechanic is greatly underrated.

After an hour of Timbo huffing and puffing, a DNS (did not start) is looking ever closer on the horizon. This is potentially a double blow. For Timbo, all the planning and training, which heavily consisted of hour-long commutes to his workplace at Brompton Hospital – Timbo has a proper job – would be wasted and for something so innocuous. Then there was the very selfish part of me that was planning to draft off Timbo the following day. (We'd completed one sportive together before, years ago. It was flat. I'd shadowed him the whole way.) I'd interviewed aerodynamicist Bert Blocken a few times and he'd measured the impact of drafting, which can provide as much as a 90 per cent energy saving in the middle of a peloton. I wouldn't have the handling skills for that but even following one rider can save up to 30 per cent energy. Basically, Timbo had to race for his sake and for mine. A step back reveals that all of this clearly isn't the end of the world. But at the time, in that situation, it seemed the most stressful thing in the world.

Incredibly, in a paroxysm of arm movements, Timbo manages to link the new chain and all is good. 'Hopefully,' says Timbo. 'I'm now a few links short so it's pretty tense.' 'Just keep off the gear extremes if you can,' I say. I'd endured similar issues when I was mountain biking and learned the hard way that as soon as the torque increased on a stiff hill, the rear derailleur and dropout snapped off. Pray for Timbo...

After the expected fitful sleep, morning arrives. And it's a positive start as the Ark is no longer needed. It's chilly but there are blue skies above. Race numbers are attached and course-profile stickers applied to the top tube. These are useful and unnerving. Useful because we can easily see where the three feed stops are placed: 30km, Velzeke; 79km, Oudenaarde; and 112km, Ronse – plus these three anchor points along the route will provide a psychological safety harness when I'm mentally dropping off a cliff. But it's equally as unnerving because the profile provides a stark reminder of the 18 climbs, or *hellingen* as locals call them, most of which are cobbled.

Bikes are reloaded and we drive the 30 minutes to Oudenaarde. The traffic system is managed well, which it needs to be as 16,000 participants have signed up for one of the most popular events on the spring sportive calendar. We park up, offload our bikes and go through the merry dance of patting ourselves front and back to check all is in order.

We're all in base layers, windproof jackets, Buffs and thick gloves. Rather splendidly, sunglasses are currently needed. Frames are loaded with two bottles each. I've gone for one electrolyte drink from Precision Hydration and one carbohydrate drink from Maurten. I stash spare powders and electrolyte tablets in my rear pockets, along with a few gels. But I keep things relatively light as I've heard the feed stations won't leave you hungry. Mini-pump packed, group selfie taken, we ride to the start line ... and away we go.

We head off together. But that bond of over 25 years – the unity forged among close friends from weddings, stag-dos, babysitting and watching sport – is instantly dismantled as we lose Kempo. To be fair, it's not unexpected. While Timbo has ticked off numerous endurance challenges, weighs nothing and cycles 800km a month, and I weigh more than nothing but have equal endurance efforts on my palmarès, this is Kempo's first organised mass event. He's actually relatively new to cycling. And, he'd admit, exercise. At university, Kempo had piled on the pounds. But recently he'd discovered Zwift and absolutely loved it. It was this that had led to the shrunken version with us today – and our decision to go bikepacking together from Ilfracombe to Plymouth in the summer of 2021. Kempo and I had enjoyed a fine weekend, despite the hangover on the Sunday, fuelled by watching England hammer Ukraine 4–0 in the European Championships the night before. That had been Kempo's first endurance challenge and he had been magnificent.

But Flanders was a different beast. There's something about pinning on the race number that fires up the competitive instinct. We soon realised that there was a split in our trio. This was in part caused by the fact that the man I called Big Man (Kempo), who's no longer the Big Man, was on a Canyon Grizl bike, which is designed for gravel. While those cobbles are jarring, a gravel bike was overkill. He'd replaced the knobbly tyres with slicks but they were still 35mm, which doesn't equate to speed. They do equate to comfort, which is what the now Middle Man (Kempo again) was after.

Timbo and I rode road bikes – Cube and Vitus. Timbo's came with 28mm tyres while mine had tubeless 25mm ones. Before signing up to Flanders, I'd not given too much mental energy to tyre selection, the premise being that life was too short. That all changed in the build-up and hammered home that even a recreational rider should adopt marginal gains when seeking not only improved performance but a cosier ride, too. (Thought logged for L'Étape du Tour in July.) After Bob Jungels had waxed lyrical about his 28s, I had put a call out to the Twitterati to gauge public opinion. I know it's anathema to the marginal gains doctrine, but unless absolutely necessary, I could do without the expense and general ball-ache of replacing a perfectly good set of tyres. The feedback was a mixed, confusing bag...

James Spragg, former professional and now top-notch coach: '25s are fine.' But... '28s are slightly better as you can run them a little softer without the danger of hitting the rim and get a bit more grip and comfort! Still, the cobbles in Flanders aren't actually that bad!'

Paul Robson: 'I did it on 25s and they were fine. Have fun. And if you have to get off on the Koppenberg, console yourself with the knowledge that the same thing happened to Merckx. I do hope you're staying for the Sunday as well (beer emoji!).'

Nick Busca: 'Did it on 25s and was good but would use 28s if I had to do it again.'

John Mc: 'They're fine. Done that on 23s back in the day. If the Koppenberg is on the parcours, try and time it so you have space as people will be getting off everywhere. If you do, get over to the side!'

And Timbo Jackson: '23s. Kempo & I need something to entertain us on the way round.'

Paralysed by choice, I do my usual and turn to my wife. 'You're overanalysing,' she says. 'Just stick with what you've got.'

She's right. I did. And I'm glad I did. By the time we arrive at the first feed station around 30km in, we've encountered two cobbled sections – the 500m Molenberg climb and the 2.3km-long but flat Paddestraat. They're like nothing I've ridden before and vibrate far more than they look like they should when viewed online, the 2D image hiding the bumps. But it's manageable. It's also early, so this could easily change.

At the feed station, we tuck into waffles and Swiss rolls, and stock up for later too. Timbo's chain is still alive but his bike computer is dead, the first victim of the cobbles. We wait for Kempo, who looks in good shape. And then we bid him farewell as we're beginning to cool down and need to get going.

We then fall into a pattern of settling into a rhythm on the road sections before it's violently disrupted on the cobbles. Gradually, I begin to fear the temporary arrows as I've spotted a trend – they direct us on to the cobbled farm tracks that usually head upwards.

Most aren't longer than 1km but with pitches reaching 10%, they really chip away. The countryside and weather are beautiful; my energy levels aren't. Neither is my seatpost. I've come to enjoy the Vitus but it has an Achilles' heel that I've become frustratingly aware of – its seat clamp design. Unlike a traditional version that clamps around the seatpost, this one requires the screw in the top tube that presses a wedge against the post to be tightened. Unfortunately, said mechanism isn't standing up to the combination of the vibrations and my weight, as when I put the torque down – needed on the steeper pitches – it sinks. Only ever so slightly but it keeps happening. It's tiring and incredibly frustrating. No matter how many times I dismount, raise the saddle and tighten the clamp, it won't stop. Rhythm is lost. As is my good mood.

Come the second feed station at 79km, fatigue has kicked in and those vibrations are beginning to take their toll. Where the early cobbles actually seemed to refresh the legs in a massage kind of way, now it's about the aches and pains. That applies to the upper body, too. Even Timbo's beginning to feel his lower back. As for the Middle Man, I've no idea. But hopefully he's OK.

After refilling out bottles, we're off again. We kept feeding to a minimum at the second feed station as one of the great climbs of Flanders is only 4km away – the Koppenberg. Its reputation is down to quality over quantity as it's only 500m long but averages a gradient of 13% and a peak gradient of 22%. It also narrows, meaning as a couple of the Twitterers fed back to me, walking is often unavoidable with so many cyclists fighting for the same space. And so the prophecy comes true as halfway up, space is squeezed, my saddle drops and I dismount. With no chance of momentum to restart at this angle, I walk to the top. Timbo has kindly waited – if only because he has the Allen key!

For me, that's where the day really began. Despite trying to follow the guttering advice of keeping to the widths and the smoother channels, the cobbles and pitches take their toll. I'm experiencing a dip that Mark Beaumont once told me he called 'the psychological arc'. Mark holds the record for cycling around the world, completing the 29,000km route in less than 79 days. 'But distance doesn't matter,' he continued. 'Whether you ride 50 miles, 100 miles or 1000 miles, the psychological arc is the same. You start fresh, dip in the middle and at the end you perk up again. The mind and body become inseparable.'

He's right, albeit it's more of a roller-coaster to the final feed station. There, it's a brief respite before the final push. Unfortunately, that proved literal on the final climb – the notorious Paterberg. This followed the infamous Oude Kwaremont, where both Niki Terpstra and Alberto Bettiol had shaken off their rivals to win solo into Oudenaarde in 2018 and 2019, respectively. The pros climb the Kwaremont three times but, thankfully, we only had to face it once. It's over 1km long, averages a gradient of 4.2% and maxes out at 11%. It proved manageable. Just. Unlike the Paterberg. With an average gradient over 12% and a peak of over 20%, it's brutal. It may be 500m long but those are 500 very long metres. Fatigue and a sinking saddle conspire to see me dismount halfway up. Timbo digs deep and makes it all the way. Chapeau.

Again, he waits. Again, I sort out my saddle. But the worst is done. We ride to the finish. Timbo puts in a last-minute sprint. I do similar but can't match him. We've ridden for around six and a half hours but another hour can be added for fuel stops. It's been a brute of ride, which I analyse on TrainingPeaks while we're waiting for the Middle Man, Kempo, who arrives sometime later, knackered but smiling. The grey clouds have formed but the mood is light. That 144km distance comprised 2136m of climbing of which the majority was cobbles. My heart rate averaged 139bpm, though that was softened slightly by the fuel stops. I maxed out at 173bpm, which was either on the Paterberg or when cursing that damn seatpost clamp. Maximum speed was 64.7km/h, reached near the end where much of it is thankfully downhill before the Kwaremont. Average speed was 21.2km/h.

What does this mean for L'Étape du Tour? Well, I'd prefer that average heart rate to drop slightly, while either maintaining power output or slightly increasing it. If I keep following coach Phil Mosley's progressive plan and the physiological adaptation of higher aerobic capacity, increased fat burning and the capacity to sustain higher wattage for longer should happen. My weekly longer rides are increasing and the intense efforts are becoming more intense. I'm feeling fitter than I have for a few years, the long rides seem to be having an impact, and I've experienced the stress of an international event and how to manage it. Those Alpine mountains are looming larger on the horizon, but my reduced bulk is looming less, which is all rather positive.

We drive back to 'Lucinda' after playing find-the-car. Any thoughts of hitting the Gent nightlife are banished by tiredness. That tiredness also means we eat awfully again, textbook recovery nutrition of protein and carbs replaced by three bags of crisp and three bottles of beer. Arguably, it sets the template for our food consumption during the following day's pro race. We're up early and catch the train from Gent back to Oudenaarde. We ponder joining the masses on the Koppenberg or Kwaremont, where reportedly a shuttle bus can take you. But we're done. We plant ourselves outside a bar and find the weakest drink we can – the 6% Kwaremont. Needless to say, we don't move until we stagger to the finish later in the day to watch van der Poel win on the big screen. The dangerous combination of lethargy and leglessness means we're dancing in a bar by 5 p.m. and eating a kebab by 8 p.m., just after finishing our game of spot-the-puffer-jacket. (Every male cycling fan in Belgium wears one.) A very quiet train to 'Lucinda' is soon followed by bed. We wake, tired, hungover but with memories that'll live forever. (Well, memories from the Saturday. Sunday is a bit of a haze.)

6

The Race of Truth

T-minus three months

'I don't think we're making a mannequin of you just yet but we can do that. Look in the room downstairs and we have mannequins of various athletes in dismembered states. There's an Alex Dowsett [former British hour record holder], an Alistair Brownlee [two-time Olympic gold medallist in triathlon] and several others.'

I thought I'd entered the Silverstone headquarters of Vorteq Sports, one of the most progressive, high-performance companies in the country. Instead, it seems I've inadvertently strolled into *Westworld*. I'm expecting Yul Brynner to start slinging his gun any minute now. 'It might be worth making one of you down the line,' says physiologist, not android, Jamie Pringle, who is director of science and technical development at the R&D outfit. 'We all know that this level of detail can make or break a race.'

It's mid-April and I'm here to uncover just how this small British company is leading the aerodynamic arms race in professional cycling and to see what I can apply to my own performance in the build-up to the Étape. Their victim – subject – is Lawson Craddock of Team BikeExchange. Vorteq is the Australian WorldTour outfit's human-performance partner, charged with identifying the most marginal of gains via a range of cutting-edge equipment and industry-leading experts. I'm here to shadow him for the day. (I'd benefitted from the experience of bike-fitter Phil Burt [*see* Chapter 2] but this is next-level, high-tech stuff. I'd also focused on comfort with my favourite Cornishman whereas this was all about cheating drag.)

'This will be my first time seeking a more aerodynamic position in the wind-tunnel,' reveals Craddock with a Texan drawl that should come with a slingshot. 'You'll enjoy it but there's much to do before then,' says Pringle.

Craddock's body will be manipulated by various scientists over a long day of analysis, tweaking and coffee, so it's relevant to get to know 'the puppet' – Lawson's words, not mine. Lawson Craddock is 30 years old. He hasn't informed his face of this fact as he looks about 18, despite a professional career in the cut-throat world of road cycling that stretches back to 2011 and his debut with Continental team Trek-Livestrong, now Hagens Berman Axeon. He moved to Giant–Shimano in 2014, followed by another move to the team that he became synonymous with, Cannondale, in 2016, where he remained until a 2022 move to Team BikeExchange.

Once mooted as a future Grand Tour challenger, third at the now-disbanded Tour of California in 2014 proved his best general classification (GC) result. He actually garnered more column inches after crashing badly on the opening stage of the 2018 Tour de France, which resulted in a hairline fracture of his scapula. He was the last rider to cross the finish line, blood streaming down the left side of his face. Needing motivation to continue through the pain, he took to social media to announce that he'd donate $100 for every stage he finished, to rebuild Houston's Alkek Velodrome, which had been ruined by Hurricane Harvey. A GoFundMe page was set up for fans to make donations and it proved the perfect dangling carrot as Craddock made it all the way to Paris, finishing the race as the 'lantern rouge' and becoming the first rider in history to hold last place for the entire three weeks. In the process, he raised over $250,000 for the cause.

Like many riders before him, Craddock recalibrated his GC ambitions and now performs the dual role of domestique and time trial specialist, the latter seeing him win the US National Time Trial Championships in 2021 and being the reason why his team are investing in this day with Vorteq.

This is third time lucky for Craddock and me, Covid having postponed the previous two efforts to meet up. 'We will get there,' BikeExchange's performance director, Marco Pinotti, assured me over email. 'And it will be worth it. We were in the tunnel with Simon Yates and Matteo Sobrero earlier in the season and had some interesting results. That said, both enjoyed very few gains. Yates has been in the wind-tunnel many times before. This was Matteo's first visit but he has time trial in his blood and has naturally reached optimum position through many years of trial and error. He holds a great position and can generate huge power.' Which is how he came to win the 2021 Italian National Time Trial Championships and so secure a move to BikeExchange from Astana–Premier Tech.

'My next time trials are at the upcoming Giro d'Italia,' Craddock says. 'I hope to do well there but my bigger goal is the nationals toward the end of June in Tennessee. It's in a small town called Knoxville. It's around 34km long but is multiple laps of a course that's around 3km in length that has one steep hill in the middle. It'll be a good one [at which] to have dialled-in aerodynamics.'

I ask Craddock who his domestic rivals will be in 'The Race of Truth', as the Giro d'Italia is sometimes dubbed. '[Magnus] Sheffield [of Ineos Grenadiers], for sure. He's young [20] so you never know if he can hold form all year but he should be strong. There's also Chad [Haga], though he's dropped down to ProSeries racing this year...' That's second division. 'And maybe Joey [Rosskopf], who races for the same team [Human Powered Health].'

Winning any national championship is clearly a major achievement but US racing these days seemingly lacks the depth of Lance Armstrong and Floyd Landis' heyday. Jumbo–Visma's Sepp Kuss and EF Education–EasyPost's Neilson Powless are outstanding riders, but only UAE Team Emirates' Brandon McNulty looks capable of becoming the USA's next cycling superstar. But he's 24 and has Tadej Pogačar ahead of him. If he's to graduate to the next level, arguably he'll have to move. 'Yeah, road cycling's not so popular in the US at the moment,' Craddock reflects. 'We just don't have professional road races, which is a shame. There are a ton of gravel events but road racing's taken a big hit.'

Presumably the positive Lance effect has flipped since confessing all to Oprah. Craddock's fellow Texan would have loved today's aerodynamic audit though, his obsession with gains not always illegal. And it starts via a stretch-and-learn session with chartered physiotherapist Bianca Broadbent. I'd come across Broadbent before at the now-closed Boardman Performance Centre. She has a calm, authoritative demeanour and voice that reminds me of my youth and artist-cum-TV-presenter Tony Hart. She could tell you your house is on fire, children have been kidnapped or the bike's been nicked (again) and her soft, velvety tones would soften the blow.

Craddock, in team bib shorts and casual T-shirt, sits on a stool like a naughty schoolboy while Broadbent runs through a series of performance and health questions, writing the answers on a whiteboard with a big black marker.

'Any issues with feet?'

'I do experience stabbing pains around the toe area when it's hot. I use a metatarsal pad and that kind of helps.'

Note to one's self: I have something in common with a world-class cyclist.

'Can you hold your current aero position comfortably?'

'For the most part, yeah. At the nationals I'll be riding for around 40 to 45 minutes. I can keep a pretty streamlined position for that time, averaging around 400 to 450 watts with a cadence of about 100rpm.'

Further note to one's self: I have very little in common with a world-class cyclist.

Broadbent then asks Craddock about previous injuries. This could take a while. Professional cyclists and injuries are unhappy bedfellows. For an article in *Cyclist* back in late 2014, I flew with photographer Juan Trujillo Andrades to Gran Canaria to interview and photograph cycling's then hottest property, Tinkoff–Saxo's Peter Sagan. We recced locations in which to photograph the Slovakian the next day before coming across the team's communications director Pierre Orphanidis. 'Unfortunately, we can't have photos of Peter in his Tinkoff kit go public until 1 January 2015,' he explained. 'He's contractually obliged to wear Cannondale apparel until 31 December

2014.' The subterfuge wasn't helped by Danish journalists stalking team boss Bjarne Riis over historic doping allegations. One small soulless hotel room wasn't a great backdrop for photos. But it worked thanks, akin to Hooper and Quint in *Jaws*, Sagan lifting his top and describing his bodily war wounds with an open mix of pain and pride. 'This one on my right hip is from the Sardinian stage of the 2013 Tour. Another one on my wrist is from racing in Italy at U23 level. And this one's real good.' He pointed to his forearm to reveal a trail of lighter scarred skin against his all-year tan. A crash at the 2010 Tour Down Under left him needing 18 stitches.

In short, even the most dexterous of athletes is lucky to avoid the pitfalls of riding at 70km/h in the peloton, with a study in the *British Journal of Sports Medicine*[10] suggesting a pro suffers from 1.2 injures each year. The most common injury is abrasions (63 per cent) followed by contusions (23 per cent) – or scrapes and bruises in common parlance. Further research in the *Orthopaedic Journal of Sport Medicine*[11] examined injury rate at the Tour de France between 2010 and 2017. Among the 1584 cycling entries evaluated over the eight-year study, 259 cyclists withdrew: 138 of those were down to acute trauma, 49 per cent of which were fractures, with the clavicle being the most commonly fractured bone. Professional cycling is a dangerous game.

'I've fractured my wrist and sternum, separated both shoulders, and currently have a fractured metacarpal [a bone that connects the fingers to the hand and wrist] and bruised ribs from a crash about a month ago,' Craddock says.

'You're going to need another whiteboard,' Pringle jests. 'But what Bianca's doing is understanding the interaction between the physical and the technical. Find out the performance history for future performance trajectory. She's painting a picture, which we'll take into the tunnel later. What do we need to look at? What don't we need to look at? Where are the challenges and opportunities – which are sometimes one and the same?'

By the end of the assessment, Bianca's 'Problem List' features that stabbing pain; whether his 172.5mm-long cranks are the right size for his 1.78m frame; if his Giant saddle's suitable for longer time trials; and maintaining high power output in the aero position under fatigue.

'Now, touch your toes,' Bianca orders. Craddock does as he's asked, effortlessly. I can touch my ankles and promise myself every year I'll take up Pilates. I will definitely do so in 2023… 'You're really flexible in the spine,' says Bianca. 'Now squat one-legged and go as low as you can. Decent. How much do you stretch?'

'I never stretch,' Craddock replies. Excellent – I'll hold that Pilates membership till 2024. This feels an opportune moment to reflect on my off-the-bike work. Mosley's plan featured a weekly strength-and-conditioning (S&C) session to reduce injury and improve flexibility, the latter of which would have been particularly useful off the back of Phil Burt's stiff-hip revelation in Chapter 2. But while I'd been committed-ish to the physio ball, the same can't be said of the S&C and mobility efforts. As you'll see in my Training Notes (Appendix 1, p. 252), I dabbled at the start of the plan but was simply too squeezed with work, life and the universe to fit everything in. 'If you drop one session, make it one of those,' Phil had told me. 'It's good to get as much time on the saddle as possible.' So that was that. S&C work banished. How that'd affect me in France, time would tell. But I am taking great joy in Craddock's confession. That said, his right-leg single-squat's not quite as impressive and Bianca mentions there are loads of Brit physios out in Craddock's European base of Girona.

'There's a massive expat community over there,' interrupts Ben Day, Craddock's trainer, who's added some colour to the day via a jaunty straw hat with single feather poking out. Australian Day raced professionally for 14 years and specialised in time trial, winning his national championships in 2003 and finishing second at the Commonwealth Games three years later. 'Lot of athletes do yoga over there,' he continues. 'It's the same in Boulder [Colorado]. I lived there for 10 years and everyone's a fucking world champion. They'd all be doing yoga. So, I tried it. But they'd all be doing handstands and I couldn't even touch my toes.'

Broadbent then feels she's heard a slight clicking sound in Craddock's right knee. She looks off into the distance, computes and then back at Craddock. 'I think you might have injured your lateral collateral ligament at some point. There's a little instability. You might have had it for years but once it's gone, it's gone. It's not really an issue for cycling but maybe keep it on your radar for the end of season.'

'Do you do any running,' Bianca asks? 'Fuck no,' Craddock retorts. So, no following Mr Armstrong's short-lived route into Ironman triathlon (until he was banned for his cycling misdemeanours) once he's retired. 'It's strange because I usually crash on my left side, though I do remember a crash around 12 or 13 years ago where I landed on my bike and since then, if I'm playing tennis, I'd have a stabbing pain in my glute.'

'Hmmm, that might link to knee stability as your hip and knee would have to work harder,' Bianca muses. 'You could even have done it as a kid. I had one female athlete undergo PCL [posterior cruciate ligament] construction. All her life she felt her knee was unstable and the only thing she could attribute it to was falling down the stairs when she was three. But it's really nothing to worry about unless you're into pivot sports.'

Craddock explains how he plays basketball in the off-season and is mildly concerned that this could spell the end of his b'ball days. Bianca says it all should be good. And anyway, there's little time to worry about that as it's now time for him to hop on to the Wattbike. That's the cue for engineer Ellis Pullinger to finish fiddling with Craddock's Giant Trinity.

Bianca tells Lawson to take it steady at around 95rpm. He'll then stick at a certain wattage while the Vorteq team run their eyes and scanning equipment over his lower limbs and upper-body position. It's a similar set-up to my session with Phil Burt but less sweaty and more about marginal gains than maximal ones.

'Right, put those hands and elbows together,' instructs Bianca. 'How narrow can those shoulders go? Can you scrunch your shoulders? We'll play around with bars and see how you react…'

Bianca is aiming to present a narrower rather than lower Craddock profile. This is a relatively recent development as in years gone by it was all about reducing the frontal profile on the longitudinal plane (in layman's terms, getting as low and flat as possible). Now, it seems, it's more about squeezing the lateral plane, as Pinotti reminded me over email. 'When I raced professionally [1998–2013], it was about getting very low, certainly in the early 2000s. Now, the trend's to tilt the bars up around 10° and close to the chin.'

Ineos Grenadiers' rider-cum-performance-engineer Dan Bigham is a master of aerodynamics. In 2021, he increased Sir Bradley Wiggins' 54.526km/h record to 54.723km/h. Though Bigham didn't use a power meter during the record, he calculated that he averaged around 350 watts. That's impressive but around 100 watts fewer than Wiggins' 450-watt hour effort. Despite that, his bullet-like profile was slick enough to overcome any wattage shortfall.

To put that into Craddock perspective, the American says that when he finished sixth in the time trial category at the 2019 UCI Road World Championships in Yorkshire, he averaged around 400 watts for over 65 minutes. Had his drag-reducing set-up been more like Bigham's than Wiggins', he would have threatened the podium, if not the gold medal.

It's why Pringle and Craddock are locked in bar talk over the whirring of the Wattbike. 'We had your teammate, Luke [Durbridge], in here recently and he had a set of customised bars from Sync Ergonomics,' Pringle says. 'I use off-the-shelf bars,' Craddock replies with a hint of envy. 'Luke's were moulded to him and his contact points, to the extent that I couldn't squeeze my arms into the arm cups,' Pringle continues. 'We have an option to design similar for you. I think Luke's were around three or four grand but they really help cut drag. Then again, high-sided cups like Luke's might not work for you. It's stuff like that we'll discover more about in the wind-tunnel.'

Craddock continues to pedal away to nowhere on the static bike but his mind is elsewhere. While the Vorteq team look at saddle pressure and the importance of insoles and play around with numerous iterations of bar positioning, Craddock's ready to be blasted in front of a turbine. Thankfully, it's tunnel time.

'OK, grab a spot of lunch, take a breather and we'll head over to the tunnel,' says Pringle. 'This is the fun part.' And the more expensive part, with the Aero Power package, which includes six hours of assessment and wind-tunnel time, costing £1275. To be honest, I'd expected it to be more as this is cutting-edge stuff from world-class practitioners.

Around £200 an hour for differences that can make or break careers seems positively frugal. Not just careers, in fact, but bragging rights.

'We have a lot of amateur time triallists come in,' says Pullinger as he eases into his cockpit overlooking the wind-tunnel. 'They're actually streets ahead of the professionals because they're not restricted as much by UCI regulations [such as those relating to tube widths, aerobar length, the saddle position, etc.]. On the WorldTour you also have sponsor obligations [meaning you can't, for example, just plunder a more aerodynamic wheel from a rival brand]. The difference between an entry-level and top-end time trial bike can be five grand and save you a handful of watts. Or you could have a more affordable wind-tunnel session and save 30 watts. I'd know which one I'd choose.'

And I know which one Craddock will choose. He's slipped into his current skinsuit, a striking stars-and-stripes form-fitting number in recognition of his 2021 US time trial triumph. His accoutrements include a stubby aero helmet, designed to cut drag, and overshoes, also designed to cut drag. He's on his Giant time trial bike, which is, you guessed it, designed to cut drag. There's an equipment theme here but today's more about positional wattage savings than trying new gear. Hence, there will be many bar-positional changes that'd be imperceptible to most but noticeable to both Craddock and Pringle, whose excitement levels have matched, if not eclipsed, the American's. 'This is my church,' he (doesn't) say, 'and tonight God is an aerodynamicist.'

Pringle explains, 'Positional changes are less about making the numbers smaller but [more] about putting him in a position that allows him to stay in that position for a longer time. We saw that with Simon. Even though the aero numbers weren't smaller, it resulted in an overall faster position.

'With Lawson we don't quite know what the optimum balance between aerodynamics and biomechanics [will be] but Bianca's given me a list of things to consider. Sometimes it's clear cut, sometimes not. In this case we need to identify what's the best posture and reverse engineer it.'

It's a positional Rubik's Cube. You sort one side and notice things have gone awry on the other. When Craddock goes wider, his upper body squares off, resulting in a narrower position overall. But frontal area, adds Broadbent, is just one aspect. That might improve numbers upfront but it might change the flow of air around his hips, meaning he's actually less aerodynamic.

'A lot of this is counter-intuitive,' Pullinger interrupts. 'Bianca and I both race and, as you can see, we're both very skinny. You'd think that might produce really great aero numbers but we're like parachutes. It's because our bones protrude and we have lots of sharp edges. Also, my arms aren't actually big enough to maximise the benefits of some fabrics, which depend on speed, size, shape and position. There are different fabrics for different scenarios. Skinny people have fewer options. Basically, tall, skinny people are the worst. If you're bigger, you fill in those gaps in-between better.'

So there you have it, 45 years of gradual gluttony has engineered my torso and limbs into an aerodynamicist's dream. Maybe I didn't need to bother with all that rather tiring Étape du Tour training nonsense, after all…

In the background, the wind-tunnel is now on and running at 50km/h. Craddock is in place and has adopted his aero position and will cycle for short increments. He will continue to do this for over an hour, with Pringle ever so slightly altering the bar position, whether by height or width, forwards or back, before rushing back to his cockpit to join Pullinger and check the data.

'We have three cameras upfront and four rear view cameras,' Pringle says. 'Lawson's key brief is to look where he would for a time trial. Not head down, not head right up. Straight ahead.' Pringle speaks into his mike and tells Craddock he's going great, then he looks back at the room. 'It's time to play CdA Bingo.'

A brief physics lesson is necessary here. CdA is the rider's coefficient of drag. Aerodynamic drag is air resistance attributed to an object. That figure is a product of an object's drag coefficient (Cd), or 'slippiness', and its size – in particular, its frontal area (A). Drag is simply those two figures multiplied.

CdA ranges upwards of zero. Physics dictates that an object with a drag coefficient 0 can't exist on Earth. Something that is very much real are teardrop-shaped bars, which can register a drag coefficient figure of 0.005. That's aero. A brick might be 2.0. Not surprisingly, that's not aero. CdA examples of elites using aero-shaped bars might come in at the 0.18–0.25 mark. For a good amateur athlete, that'd be more like 0.25–0.30.

'What do you think, Ben?' Pringle repeats, warming to his game 'I reckon 0.28,' he replies. 'Better than that – 0.213.'

'Right, I think we're done for now,' Pringle says. And the result? 'Lawson is aerodynamically stubborn. By that I mean there's a reason why he's wearing that stars-and-stripes suit – he's good. Very good. The bigger changes will come via a faster skinsuit and different overshoes.' And with that, a chap brandishing what looks like a '90s camcorder enters the control room.

This is George from Catesby Innovation Centre, who like Vorteq sit beneath the aerodynamic umbrella of Northamptonshire-based company TotalSim. 'This is a fancy video camera that captures 30 frames a second,' he explains. 'It takes standard visible light photos but projects an infrared grid. We're going to map Lawson and create his own suit.'

And with that, George enters the tunnel, the light goes out, there's a flash to briefly reveal Lawson and then it's dark again. 'I'm done,' says George. And he's off.

'With that data of Lawson's body, we'll source specialist materials and, thanks to four seamstresses who work here, we'll stitch Lawson a suit,' says Pringle. This is arguably Vorteq's USP, resulting in some head-turning results. At the following month's Giro, Simon Yates won his first-ever Grand Tour time trial wearing a bespoke Vorteq suit that cost around £3500.

'The flow of air over surfaces is speed sensitive,' adds Pringle. 'Something that works at 50km/h doesn't work at 65km/h. That's because airflow changes according to speed regarding where air separates and becomes turbulent. It's how you control that flow that's important. That's a challenge and that's where the money goes: understanding those dynamics. It's why some of the tech in here I could tell you about but [then] I'd have to kill you.

'It's why Alex Dowsett's hour-record suit was different on one side than the other,' Pringle continues. 'In the velodrome, you're always turning to your left. As you lean, you experience an acceleration of flow over one side, which is effectively a yaw angle. That leads to different airflow on either side and is why the suit he used was asymmetric.'

Could this course-specific suit idea be taken to the more dynamic open roads of a race like the Tour de France, I ask? 'Well, you could have the directeurs sportifs drive a couple of hours ahead of the lead rider and determine wind conditions. They do that for wheel selection but you could do that for clothing too. The ideal would be you'd have 20 suits for various different course and wind conditions and choose based on that. That might sound unrealistic but it could happen. Their importance is understated by many. In track cycling, we've seen some huge wattage gains and this is at 80km/h. Riders have gone from fifth in qualifying to qualifying fastest.'

So progressive is Vorteq's clothing that the Smithsonian Museum in Washington D.C., USA, has Ashton Lambie's suit on display. 'He broke the four-minute barrier for 4000m wearing that suit and I designed it,' says Pullinger, beaming. 'I chose all the custom fabrics and fine-tuned it.'

Craddock will hope for similar gains as he wipes down and Pringle mops up. 'Right, we'd better head off as we have a flight to catch,' says jaunty-hatted Day.

It's been an enlightening day, highlighting how even a mid-40s male with fatty deposits (though fewer than in January) can improve aerodynamics. One of the key take-homes is regarding positioning. In France, I'll be aboard my Vitus road bike, so this time-trial tinkering won't be needed. But I can certainly spend greater time on the drops. Traditionally, I'm a drops-atheist, believing that the tops or hoods (both parts of the bar that leave you more upright) are home for my clammy hands. The drops, well, those entail a more bent-over position that I've never felt I could sustain. In all honesty, the S&C and mobility work that I'd sacrificed could have helped here, but even without that, simply cycling so consistently and for so many hours has strengthened my core, making the more aerodynamic drops a place that I could commit to frequenting more regularly. Not for the full Étape du Tour, of course, that'd be crazy talk, but for downhills and easy stretches of flat road – please tell me there are easy stretches of flat road! – the drops certainly offer the topography that might enable me to save a little time.

Two months later, in June, I'm after a Craddock update in terms of both position and performance. He's completed the sixth Grand Tour of the eight he's started, finishing 107th. That overall placing is irrelevant as Craddock was at the Giro d'Italia in service of Simon Yates, who would abandon on stage 17 because of persistent knee issues. Team BikeExchange did, however, win both time trials thanks to Yates and Matteo Sobrero, rewarding the work of Pinotti, Day and the Vorteq team.

'I gave both time trials a good crack but the end result wasn't what I expected,' Craddock tells me over phone from his sweltering Texan home. 'The first time trial [in which he placed 156th] was incredibly technical. I think after having kids [Lawson has two], you lose a little of that fearless factor. I felt great but lost time in 21 turns. On the final time trial [in which he placed 36th] on the last day, I was feeling the three weeks in my legs and lost time on the descent.'

That opening time trial, in particular, is no gauge of Craddock's abilities. Day had told me in the tunnel that he wouldn't ride hard in the prologue because of his supporting role. Craddock says he's now playing around with his elbows and shoulders in search of small gains and that very minor tweaks are no bad thing. 'It gives you confidence that you have a good position. Of course, you always want insane gains and want to get your CdA down to 0.17 or 0.18. But it's not possible for everyone. Ultimately, I know it won't be the position that'll hold me back.'

It certainly didn't in Knoxville in late June, where Craddock retained his US national time trial crown, conquering the 34.9km course in 40.39 minutes at an average speed of 51.513km/h. Magnus Sheffield finished four seconds behind, with George Simpson in third. And all this Craddock achieved while squeezed into his bespoke suit. Vorteq's PR team must be delighted.

'Nothing says cool like a middle-aged man, bit of Coldplay and a spot of fake tan.' So rapped 47-year-old Paul Alborough, aka Professor Elemental, the steampunk and 'chap-hop' musical artist that my mate Timbo had insisted I listen to en route back from Gent. I'm glad I did. He's brilliant. Surreal, silly and satirically spot on. The lyrics are swirling around my rather large cranium as I look in the mirror. 'Not bad,' I nod to myself. 'A few lumps and bumps but better than several months back.'

A grand-plus wind-tunnel session is beyond my budget but there are positional, gear and clothing ideas from my Craddock day that I can more affordably integrate into my Étape du Tour journey. It's why I'm currently in a Scott trisuit that I've dug out from the deepest, darkest depths of my 'sports drawer'. A place where run shorts, bib shorts, cycle tops, compression socks, post-event T-shirts, the occasional event medal, winter clothing, summer clothing and much more besides wrestle for space. Tonight, I'm to 'race' a time trial in nearby Dursley, Gloucestershire, the twofold aim being to test my fitness beyond the laboratory and the Wattbike, plus it's what the pros do. As I'm on my no-pro journey, I don't really have a choice. I'm deep into Mosley's training plan and I'm feeling stronger and a little lighter. I'm feeling quite good about myself, until my wife walks in. 'I never need to see you in that again.'

'Nothing says fool like a middle-aged man in Lycra...'

It could be worse. I'd recently interviewed Rob Lewis. Lewis is the founder of TotalSim, the company behind Vorteq. His aerodynamic palmarès is huge and includes being a core member of British Cycling's Secret Squirrel Club, which formed in 2004 to drive innovation. Chris Boardman was the highest-profile Squirrel. Lewis said they'd managed to cut around 12 per cent drag from many of the track riders in the build-up to the 2008 Olympics by manipulating the airflow and cutting drag via clothing advancements. It was a game changer and contributed to Team GB winning 14 medals in the Beijing velodrome, eight of which were gold. He also mentioned that nothing was off-limits during the development phase, including a rider's dignity, though thankfully not all of these came to fruition. 'We created sequin suits and ones with fur impregnated in places, all designed to improve aerodynamics. We even talked about selective shaving or plaiting the hairs on legs. We had plenty of wacky ideas.'

'I might like you in a sequin skinsuit,' my wife comments with a smile. Or smirk. Help.

But back to my outing today. Britain arguably has a stronger time trial heritage than road racing, producing some of our country's best riders, including Beryl Burton, Sir Bradley Wiggins, Chris Boardman and Graeme Obree. Its roots lie in a decision made in 1890. While the rest of mainland Europe was beginning to bunch ride on this relatively new invention called a bicycle, the National Cyclists' Union, the forerunner to today's British Cycling, banned all cycle racing on public roads – a ban that ran until the 1950s. Why this was so is not 100 per cent certain though the story goes, apocryphal or not, that there was an 'incident' between a lady, her horse and a group of cyclists. For safety's sake, all future events would have to be held on the track.

This didn't go down well, sending the racers underground. Rebel riders would meet at dawn, at clandestine locations only known by code and dressed entirely in black. They would set off solo a couple of minutes apart and race the clock rather than each other. That way, if the police were to stop a rider, they could say they were just out for a gentle spin. The first of these illicit time trials was reportedly held in North London in 1895 and run by the North Road Cycling Club. An act intended to improve safety had inadvertently spawned an integral part of modern cycling.

Time trialling has long gone overground but its appeal and absurdity remains. It's why once I'd left my wife pondering divorce, I'm parked up next to Chapel Hill Business Park between Newport and Woodford with a group of around 20 equally compressed, but less alarming-looking, individuals ready to ride as fast as we can down a stretch of the A38 that links Bristol to Gloucester. There are cars whizzing past at 97km/h, people waiting at a bus stop, all while riders with teardrop helmets, visors, time trial bars and all manner of aerodynamic wizardry sign up to tonight's proceedings, run from the car boot of one of Dursley Road Club's (DRC) committed members.

Some events require membership but this is a 'Come and Try It' event for non-members like me. Tonight is the club's 10-mile offering. That's a common TT distance, as is the 25-miler. Tonight's efforts will cost me the grand total of £6. For DC members, it's £3.50. This is no commercial money-making operation, which is another part of the appeal.

This'll be the first club-organised road event I've ever tackled, which I guess is hardly surprising as I'm not a member of a cycling club. 'Had I thought of joining a club for your training,' you might ask? No. Which sounds abrupt and I might have been missing a trick, but I did have three solid(ish) reasons why. The first is I wanted to follow Mosley's plan to the letter. I could do that solo; in a group, that wouldn't happen. Second, I felt joining a club and the extra social side that brings, plus writing about cycling, plus training for L'Étape du Tour would be too much cycling. I love this sport but it can't be everything. I need more than that, which arguably is one of the many reasons I never made it as an elite sportsman. Finally, though a sociable fellow at times, often I'm more than happy with my own company. Hence why I'm a writer, I guess.

'It sounds strange to say it but I enjoy meeting in a lay-by and having a bit of a social,' DRC member Andy Muitt tells me beside the bins beside the industrial estate beside the traffic. I was right – don't join a club. They're crazy dudes! 'Some people, of course, can't think of anything worse than going up and down an A-road. It's an individual thing, though when you explain it to others, granted it sounds a little weird. But when you're doing it, as you'll find out, you're not thinking about the A-road. You're just in your own little zone thinking, can I go faster?'

If I can't, it won't be for want of trying. Beyond racking up more training miles than I've ever ridden before and beyond my form-fitting indecent exposure, I'm wearing a set of polyester arm warmers. It's a balmy evening but I've taken on board advice from Vorteq's engineer Ellis Pullinger, who said wearing them was an easy win, especially if you have drag-inducing hairy arms. I am, however, not using clip-on tribars, the reason being that I want this to give me feedback for the Étape about holding a position on the drops, especially on the descents. And, of course, I don't currently own a pair. The same applies to my helmet. It's a vented road bike helmet for god knows how many hot hours in France, rather than an aero one. Other gear that'll project me through the Dursley air are a pair of Look pedals and an 11-speed electric groupset from Shimano. Neither is aerodynamic but they do make me more efficient. That groupset in particular is rather fun, the reassuring whirring sound with each shift reminding me I'm really just a large boy with an innovative toy. I have a mild concern that while I have plenty enough gears for the flats of Gloucestershire, the same might not apply to the mountains of France. It's been OK thus far around north Somerset and the Mendips, and handled Flanders – just – but changing the cassette on the rear wheel for something more attuned to steep hills is on my boys-toys radar. Whether I'll act on that radar warning remains to be seen.

As for many of the other racers, it looks like they've just rolled straight out of Silverstone. 'This? Oh, this is all old gear,' Paul Tutton of Velo Club Bristol says modestly. 'You really want a breakdown? OK, it's a Dolan Scala with 7900 Dura Ace groupset plus Rotor Q rims and ceramic jockey wheel, a Zipp Super 9 rear tubular wheel with Conti Sprinter tubs, plus Planet-X 60mm deep-section carbon front with another Conti Sprinter tub and 3T Aura Pro cockpit, while I'm wearing a Carnac Kronus Time Trial helmet complete with visor.' Tutton doesn't stop to draw breath. 'I also have a 30mm riser upfront so my beer gut doesn't hit my knees and I like Thatcher's Gold.'

This, I soon discover, is very much the double-life of the time triallist: riders, many of them older like 52-year-old Tutton, love the engineering side of things, of testing themselves, before discussing gains with like-minded folk over a pint or two. In theory, I can see the appeal. Will the same hold in practice? 'Just don't go off too fast,' Tutton continues. 'Go off like a million miles an hour for the first mile and a half and you'll pay for it.'

I might also pay for a supplementary decision I'd made, as I thought I'd give sodium bicarbonate a go. Yes, baking powder, albeit I ordered it in pill form as I didn't think it would feel as odd, or disgusting, as spooning myself several grams of the white stuff.

Why had I just topped up Jeff Bezos' bank account once more with said purchase? Well, a few years ago I had attended an edition of the Science & Cycling Conference in France, where I had come across Dr Andy Sparks, an exercise physiology specialist at Edge Hill University, Lancashire. 'In a series of experiments, we showed that you can enjoy an average performance improvement of 2.2 per cent in a time trial by taking sodium bicarbonate,' Sparks had said.

It's all rather ingenious and comes down to the intensity at which you ride a time trial. It's been described as a tightrope. Or as former hour record-holder Chris Boardman has often been quoted as saying, 'The key equation I had in my head was: how far is it to go and is my current pace sustainable? If the answer is yes then you're not going hard enough, if the answer is no then it's already too late, so the answer you're looking for is maybe, and that effort is totally relevant to the distance.'

In short, you're riding as sustainably hard as you can for the distance desired. Psychologically, that's brutal. Physiologically, it means you're relying more on glycogen (glucose stores) for fuel than fats. In turn, and as Dr Iñigo San-Millán explained in Chapter 4, you generate great swathes of lactic acid, which can ultimately lead to the 'burn' and a drop in power output.

Which is where sodium bicarbonate comes in. Because it's an alkaline, it raises the pH of your blood, so that when lactic acid tips over from your working muscles to your bloodstream, essentially you've got a wider acidic bandwidth before pH levels drop to a level that fatigues muscles.

So, all good? Not quite. 'The problem is that this alkaline rise often results in gastro-distress,' said Sparks. Namely, the trots. 'However, our research has shown that individualising dose and timing of sodium bicarbonate can improve performance without making the gut "too lively".'

Experienced time triallists might have played around with the standard protocol of 0.3g of sodium bicarbonate per kilogram of bodyweight ingested 60 minutes before intense exercise. 'But our studies showed this is too generic,' Sparks explained. 'For some riders, pH levels peaked after 10 minutes; others up to 90 minutes. Also, some benefitted from 0.2g; others came in at over 0.3g.'

On this night, my weight hovered around 88.5–89kg, which I was pleased about from the 92kg-plus of January. Rather dangerously, since Sparks said that 15 per cent of riders can suffer stomach issues, I went for the upper end of 0.3g, which equated to 2.6g of sodium bicarbonate. Each pill contained 500mg of the good stuff, so around an hour before the start I necked five, washed down with water. I metaphorically clenched, hoping I wouldn't literally have to do the same.

'Five, four, three, two, one...' And the first rider was off. The countdown with a flourish emanated from John Roberts, DRC member for nine years. Roberts, staring intently at his stopwatch, would set off riders every 60 seconds. With 15 seconds to go, each rider would clip into their pedals and be held upright by club legend John Sirett, who'd raced for the club since 1970. 'It used to be a school club,' the svelte 64-year-old would tell me later. 'I came home from school and told my dad I wanted to join, so I inherited his bike. It was a Viking bike used by the Viking professional team of the '50s. I've raced on and off for DRC ever since.'

He was on volunteer duty this evening but, when racing, still clocks around 24 minutes for 16km. That's impressive. As I wobbled in preparation for the off, he told me to take it easy and just aim for sub-30 minutes so I had a benchmark.

'Three, two, one...' I'm off on this gently rolling parcours. And before I know it, I'm overtaking experienced riders dressed in all sorts of aero paraphernalia. Marshals bow and curtsey as I pass and word has got around. There's a pincer movement as crowds from Gloucester, Cheltenham and Bristol descend on Dursley to catch sight of the new Wiggins scorching down the A38. Fireworks are fired and fans faint over the exhibition of speed they've just witnessed...

OK, it's not long before I'm overtaken by a rider whose CdA looks sub-0.15. I hear him before I see him, the sound of that disc wheel rising and falling as he passes. But I overtake the rider ahead – alright, I admit it, they've punctured – and soon settle into a hard but sustainable pace. Dropping the empirical for one evening, I'm riding by feel rather than power. I'm not looking to break any records. I just want to concentrate on position and enjoying it.

How much you can enjoy riding up and down a carriageway is, as Muitt said, theoretically debatable. But he was right – in practice, your world shrinks to a small imaginary box in front of you. It's more about checking in with yourself, about scrunching your shoulders, ensuring your power's good, your cadence is high and you're in the rhythm. I mix between the hoods and drops, and actually feel like I'm riding rather fast. The Scott suit and warmers might look offensive but they certainly compress, meaning there are no ripples or flapping. It means a quiet ride and, in my eyes (or ears), if it's a quiet ride, it means air resistance is down, meaning more speed.

Sirett said to take it easy but I know I've got more in me, so I crank things up a bit. I can always back down if needed. Which is actually a pacing strategy that might pay off as there is more than one way to skin a cat. While a 2012 study in the *European Journal of Applied Physiology*[12] showed that optimum speed and lower physiological stress and perceived exertion come from an even pacing strategy, further research in 2013[13] suggests a parabolic (U-shaped) pacing model is best. British research discovered that time triallists who started fast, eased off slightly in the middle and then upped the pace at the end enjoyed faster times, a higher average intensity and lower stress than their even-paced contemporaries. Then there's Dutch research, featured in the *International Journal of Sports Physiology and Performance*[14], which concluded that continuous variations in pace could actually hold the secret to maximum performance.

That Dutch study was particularly interesting as although they weren't 100 per cent sure why this was the case, they suggested it might be down to Professor Tim Noakes' Central Governor Model of Fatigue[15], which says that effort is tightly regulated by the brain, rather than any chemical change in the muscle. Let me explain. The brain works 24/7 and is constantly processing a huge amount of physiological, emotional and environmental feedback. However, maintaining some form of homeostasis isn't a static process, it's highly dynamic. Take your hormonal profile, for example. Stress can lead to a rise in cortisol and adrenaline, leading to a fight-or-flight scenario. The brain seeks safety – it seeks levelling out of this rise and fall. But deviations happen. We're humans. Expecting us to lock in and stick rigidly to the same cadence or effort is to ignore the natural adjustments our bodies are constantly making and are programmed to want to make. Which could explain the idea that a natural rise, fall and then rise is actually an optimum process.

Back on the A38, my earlier enthusiasm is waning somewhat, the rising pain in my thighs suggesting the power I'd risen to was unsustainable. By now, though, I've 180ed the roundabout turnaround point and am on the way back, resulting in more speed for less wattage as the gentle headwind had flipped to a tailwind. And before I know it, I've crossed the finish line. Well, crossed John with stopwatch and clipboard in hand. I finish at around 28 minutes at an average speed of 34.6km/h.

That's way behind tonight's fastest ride of Tom Williams in 20 minutes and 19 seconds and even further behind the club record of one Arthur Franklin, who broke through the 48.3km/h average with a time of 19 minutes and 12 seconds. But I'm happy. I felt strong, in a good, sustainable position and there were no bicarb repercussions, though it was nigh on impossible to gauge how much it had impacted things. I'd need a far more diligent study to work that one out. But I certainly felt good.

At the WorldTour level, riders warm down on a set of rollers after an event. This is to shake off fatigue in readiness for the next day's stage and spin out lactic acid. In all honesty, I should do the same after a time trial but convince myself that with no 250km romp in the mountains to follow, I'll instead assess some of the glittering bikes on display. With that, I have my head turned by a stealth black number that looks like it's rocketed over from NASA.

'That's Bo's bike,' says Muitt. 'He's a brilliant example of a tinkerer. Me? I keep things the same most weeks. But Bo, well, it's like Formula One. He'll tweak, assess, tweak, assess.' Bo's latest tweak, which I was drawn to, was a sheet of carbon fibre between his bar extensions. 'Here he is now,' Muitt adds.

'Yeah, I added that to my Orbea Ordu,' Bo explains in his formidable West Country accent, before echoing Pullinger's sentiments about UCI and sponsorship restrictions meaning the amateur scene is in many ways more progressive. 'They'd be banned in a pro race, which is a loss to the pros as they help the airflow around your arms, especially in the narrower position that's popular now.' Bo is around 1.7m, in his mid-60s and is a powerhouse. He's dressed in a high-end NoPinz skinsuit with NoPinz overshoes. His head is streamlined thanks to an aero helmet and visor. 'Those socks would be banned, too, as they're full length. The UCI only allow three-quarter length.'

Bo and Muitt are here week in, week out, for both the competition and the craic. But that competition is against yourself, they agree. 'It doesn't matter what times you do,' Muitt continues. 'It's all about improving your own efforts. If you come first or last, you're treated as an equal. At the end of day, it's all about having fun with a great group of people.' It was and they are. Just like the cyclo-cross and the cobbled scene. My Étape challenge is looming larger on the horizon but on this rather busy carriageway, all is good with the world.

A couple of days pass and I reflect on my Vorteq–Dursley double-header. Was I feeling more confident for the research and minor application I'd undertaken? Yes and no. I'd certainly seen the aerodynamic importance of banning clothing that flaps in the wind and I'd felt strong in my Gloucestershire TT. But when observing Craddock, as interesting as it all was, I could feel myself veering into paralysis by analysis. Throw in the stress of a house move and Covid clinging on to my wife's immune system and I had to remind myself to breathe, Jimbo, breathe. And enjoy. I was in a privileged position that should raise a smile, not drag out a grimace. I was deep into my French adventure and I'd immersed myself into this vibrant, friendly and beautiful cycling community. All that said, boy did I need some rest, recuperation and repair…

7

Go and Go Again...

T-minus two and a half months

The 2022 Giro d'Italia measured 3445km, of which over 52,000m was uphill. That was tougher than the Tour de France, which came in at a genteel 3349.8km and just 49km of climbing. As a snapshot, the Giro's 172km stage four between Avola and Mount Etna, won by Bora–Hansgrohe's Lennard Kämna, racked up over 3500m of ascending; stage seven from Diamante to Potenza, won by Jumbo–Visma's Koen Bouwman, rolled out to 196km via 4300m of ascending; and the ninth stage accumulated the peak climbing metres of the entire Grand Tour at 4785m. The parcours started in Isernia and finished atop the brutal Blockhaus, one of the highest paved mountains of the Apennine range. Bora–Hansgrohe's Jai Hindley won, laying the foundations for winning the *maglia rosa*. So iconic is this limestone wonder that when Eddy Merckx established his cycle-manufacturing company, he named one of his steel steeds after the Blockhaus.

Incredibly, this vicious trio of stages comes before the first rest day – the first week is often an 'easing' into a three-week race with pain and further pain inflicted in weeks two and three, but not at the 2022 Giro d'Italia. It's why EF Education–EasyPost's Lancastrian climber Hugh Carthy is sprawled out on his hotel bed as I Zoom 'Huge' on that first rest day after his beating on Blockhaus. Hugh's nickname is 'Huge' because his name was mispronounced by a commentator at a previous Giro. He's also known for his huge efforts and ability to dig deep. He's also huge for a climber, at 1.93m, though he weighs less than 70kg. (I've hooked up with Huge as, while I'm not completing a three-week Grand Tour – thank ruddy god – I am looking to see what pro-level recuperative advice can be assimilated and absorbed into my Étape-seeking, fatigued self.)

'It wasn't ideal,' Carthy reflects in his Preston twang, not softened by spending much of the year in his mainland European base of Girona. He lost nearly four minutes on Hindley after a piercingly hot stage took its toll. 'I had a bit of a wobble on the last climb [Blockhaus], going through a bad patch for about 15 minutes. The second half of the climb is a more favourable gradient and I found a second wind. Thankfully, I didn't lose further time.

'I've learnt from the past that you must refocus and wipe the slate clean. After today, we have another six-stage block of hard racing before the next rest day. It's important to focus on the day-to-day and recover right. Do that and you'll race smarter.'

Which is why Carthy is in the supine position that all pros seek on their rest days but that are often interrupted by press conferences, anti-doping control and, of course, answering questions from big-headed journos in another country. (I refer not to my ego, which arguably is quite big, but the size of my cranium.) 'Today has been made easier because there was a short journey from the stage finish to the hotel,' Carthy says, easing his hands behind his head as if to emphasise the point. 'Often, you'll face a long bus transfer the evening before a rest day to fit in with the post-rest-day schedule. You arrive at the accommodation late, have a rushed massage, rushed dinner and hit the sack full, hot and sticky. I'm sure avoiding that helped this morning. Yesterday was as tough as it gets, really, and I expected stiff legs this morning but after 10 minutes of spinning, they woke up.'

All three Grand Tours now deviate beyond Italian, French and Spanish borders, respectively, to spread the cycling gospel. Take the 2022 Tour de France. After three stages in Denmark, where the crowds registered in their millions, the riders, support staff and race organisation had a near-1000km transfer from Sønderborg to Dunkirk for stage four. ASO, organisers of the Tour, have been accused of treating riders like dogs, most notably in 1978 when Bernard Hinault led the protests against split stages, in which riders completed a stage in the morning followed by one later in the afternoon. Even ASO realised the Danish migration was a kilometre or 1000 too far and pencilled in an extra rest day on top of the standard two.

Carthy is in surprisingly phlegmatic mood for a rider who's just plummeted down the GC. He comments that it's down to experience, that managing your emotions is key to navigating the highs and lows of a three-week stage race. I suggest it's partly down to 24 hours away from the physicality and media spotlight of racing, which Carthy doesn't dismiss when he breaks down exactly what a rest day comprises of.

'You rise in your own time, which for most of us is around nine o'clock. On a stage day, it's around seven. Breakfast is a fair bit lighter than what we'd have on a race day. Then it would be big plates of rice, maybe a three-egg omelette and a load more. This morning it was some oats, a small omelette and some fruit.

'It's good because normally it's then about packing your suitcase for a certain time to make the bus transfer to the stage start. Today was much more chilled, meaning you can chat to folk you often don't have the chance to, like the mechanics.

'We then went for a ride of around an hour and a half at an easy intensity, though we threw in a couple of climbs. This is important to keep the blood flowing and to stave off heavy legs and lethargy; you don't want to shut down completely but you don't want to overexert yourself, either.

'We stopped for a nice coffee and soft drink, rode back to the hotel and [then it] was more or less lunchtime. A light, nutritious lunch featuring a lot of salad and some good but not heavy energy. Back to hotel room, rest and catch up on things like checking the state of supplies. If you need something from the shops – toothpaste – you can ask a staff member to get it for you today. Shave your legs, shave your face. Get organised for next week. Then it was shut the blinds and get my head down for an hour's afternoon nap, till about 15 minutes ago when I knew you were going to call.

'After we're done, I'll try and get my head down again, read a bit, and switch off from racing and travelling. At five it's a massage. Bit longer than normal, maybe focusing on some areas that you haven't really had time to focus on. Then it's a check-in with the chiropractor, who'll adjust anything that needs adjusting. From there, the doctor checks your overall health. Back to your room to rest up before dinner, where we'll fuel properly for tomorrow's stage [Pescara to Jesi]. Then to bed and that's it. It goes too quickly; you really want these days to slow down.'

Arguably it's more of an audit day than a rest day with Carthy's EF support cast ensuring he replenishes energy stores, eases out muscle soreness and kips well. The importance of R&R is highlighted by a 2017 study[16] led by Jose A. Rodriguez-Marroyo, who tested seven Continental riders (the third division of international road racing) before and after the Vuelta a España to ascertain the impact fatigue has on rider performance. The septet undertook exercise tests one week before the race and, rather brutally, just one day after the 21-stage race.

After 3265km of racing, the distance of which broke down as 2 per cent time trials, 46 per cent flat and 52 per cent mountainous, the mental and physical toll was stark. The riders' average VO_2 max dropped 9 per cent from 81.8ml/kg/min to 74.4ml/kg/min (*see* Chapter 1 for more on VO_2 max). Their functional threshold power plummeted 10.3 per cent from 437.8W to 391.5W. And their maximum heart rate dipped by 6.7 per cent, from 191bpm to 179bpm.

Overall, the seven riders endured a 10 per cent physiological drop due to several reasons: difficulty in maintaining high muscle glycogen levels, a decrease in catecholamine sensitivity (exhaustion of the neuroendocrine system), a reduction of the heart's cardiac output and muscle damage – especially in the last two weeks. Who coped best? 'Cyclists with more efficient adaptation mechanisms might be more able to sustain considerably higher exercise intensities for longer periods and/or have less body stress,' the researchers concluded. This highlights the importance of managing fatigue, and that it's physically impossible to sidestep a detriment in performance.

The key is to lessen those losses via things like rest days, a balanced training plan, massage and good nutrition.

Carthy and his fellow riders have a band of experts to cure, and to a certain extent prevent, their every ache and pain. But they also utilise a piece of tech that's available to all of us: Whoop. Those of you who spend their Julys pretending to work while the Tour plays out on Global Cycling Network (GCN)/Eurosport in the background can't have failed to notice Whoop, their adverts usually featuring an EF rider resplendent in pink while they rave about how they wouldn't have progressed from paperboy or disposed of stabilisers if it weren't for this piece of wearable tech. EF rider Alex Howes features in one ad, explaining how his entire year's training will be based on Whoop data rather than a coach.

'This year, our tactics are totally Whoop driven,' says EF's head of medicine, Dr Kevin Sprouse, of Whoop's impact at the Giro. I catch up with Sprouse via Zoom on the same rest day on which I'd spoken to Carthy. 'We are nothing without Whoop,' Sprouse continues.

The Whoop cult has taken hold. 'I jest,' says Sprouse with a grin. 'But it has proved useful. As a doctor, historically I could gather data via their power meter at a race and training. That's great but means we're missing out on 20 hours a day. Those 20 hours are significant because when a rider doesn't feel right, typically they come to us with vague complaints. With this, we can monitor their recovery and health much more accurately.'

For those not obsessed with those Tour advert breaks and who don't know what I'm on about, Whoop is a wristband that monitors sleep, recovery and daily effort. Key to this physiological insight is its HRV feature – heart rate variability, which it measures via an optical sensor and logarithms. As Whoop proclaims on its website, 'This is the variance in time between beats of your heart. So, if your heart rate is 60 beats per minute, it's not actually beating once every second. Within that minute there may be 0.9 seconds between two beats and 1.15 seconds between others. The greater the variability, the more "ready" your body is to execute a high level.' It's all tied in with the nervous system. Greater variations between beats is associated with parasympathetic activity (rest and recovery); a reduction in the variations between beats is associated with sympathetic activity (fight-or-flight). If a rider wakes and HRV is very low, that could mean they're neurologically fatigued, which might alter their training content for the day.

Measuring the heart's activity to see how an athlete is faring is nothing new, but how a company chooses to present that data can be. Whoop's adverts and marketing are loaded with riders' 'strain' scores, something GCN's Dan Lloyd is particularly partial to in his punditry. This is the company's scale of 0–21 – the higher the number, the greater the strain – and is ostensibly based on heart rate data and duration.

'I use Whoop across multiple sports and one of the things that I see with riders is massive strain scores that you don't see in other sports, certainly not as frequently,' says Sprouse. 'A strain score of 13 to 14 is a moderate day. It might be going to work and then a 45-minute run at lunch. Looking back at the Etna stage, we had six guys with a score of 20.7 and two guys with 20.6. So right up there with the toughest of days. That's only 0.1 difference but at that end of the scale, it's huge, so I'm thinking maybe the riders with 20.6 were protected a little more than the others.

'The recovery score is important, too, and that's where HRV comes in again,' Sprouse adds. 'If it's around 90 per cent, that's great. Down at 60 and they're struggling to overcome a long day.' The latest version of Whoop also measures skin temperature, adding another metric feather in its data-laden cap.

EF has used Whoop since 2020 and is contracted to 2023. Only the team know how much use is based on sponsorship or practicality. In August 2021, Whoop announced it had secured $200 million in funding after the company was valued at $3.6 billion. In a sport so heavily reliant on sponsorship – there are no ticket sales and TV revenue for teams, hence the teams' names changing depending on sponsor(s) – scepticism suggests wrist-based heart rate assessment plus logarithms is far from the gold standard.

Then again, a study in the journal *Sensors*[17] that evaluated Whoop's heart rate accuracy (of their 2.0 watch) against an electrocardiogram

(ECG) machine came up favourably. I've interviewed two of the study's authors before, Shona Halson and academic editor Marco Altini, who are sleep and HRV experts, respectively. For me, that adds credibility to the study. But then I read the 'conflicts of interest' section and it transpires that one of the authors, Dean J. Millar, 'is currently sponsored by Whoop Inc... However, this sponsorship arrangement was initiated after the data were collected for this study'. It really is an independent quagmire out there.

I've worn numerous heart rate monitors over the years and still see the chest strap as the best option. Wrist-based models, which rely on lights and blood colour, are more practical but not as accurate, especially during hard bursts of effort like a stiff climb when they seemingly struggle to accurately measure sharp rises in heart rate. Changes in wrist position, such as when going from seated to standing, can also impact the validity of results, at least temporarily.

Then again, maybe my scepticism has left me short-sighted. When I spoke to Hugh Carthy after stage nine, he wallowed down in 17th on the GC. Come the finish in Verona, he'd risen to ninth, possibly fuelled by his Whoop powers of recovery.

Speed of recovery is arguably a proxy for the health of a rider, be it Huge Carthy or Huge me. The welfare of a rider is part of Sprouse's remit, like all team doctors, including my next interviewee – Dr Adrian Rotunno. Rotunno was born in Italy but grew up in South Africa, where he studied medicine and ended up at Cape Sports Medicine specialising in sports and exercise medicine. His many roles also include head of medical at Ajax Cape Town football team (now Cape Town Spurs FC), chief medical officer for the Old Mutual Two Oceans Marathon, and he is now team physician for Tadej Pogačar's UAE Team Emirates.

I've spent time with the good doctor in the past, as well as with Richard Usher at Ineos Grenadiers, Anko Boelens at Team DSM and many others. They all have one thing in common and it's not the nefarious one many of you think: they work extremely hard. They're charged with ensuring their well-paid minions – Pogačar is on a reported £5 million per year, as I mentioned earlier – remain strong enough to perform at their optimum, made uniquely harder over the past few seasons because of Covid.

Pandemic aside, their job's an unenviable one, especially in an effort to close the window on infection. 'There's something called the "open-window theory"', explains Rotunno. 'The immune system is suppressed during intense exercise load so that "window" for falling ill opens more as the Grand Tour progresses.'

It's why the chances of infection and illness spreading through a team and their eight riders are high, and also why a rider displaying symptoms like a cough and sniffling nose will end up being moved from sharing a room to being quarantined on their own.

It's not easy. Rotunno's Grand Tours are packed with 18-hour days, the outline of which the Italian South African shared with me – it's not for the faint-hearted and made my day seem positively louche in comparison. If I'm spending time with a team at the Tour, my day might comprise: 7 a.m. alarm call, shower, buffet breakfast (*see* Chapter 1 for more on the glory of the buffet!). I'll then interview a few riders and support staff while they're milling around the hotel before heading to that day's starting town. I'll hop into one of the team cars – usually with a directeur sportif and mechanic – and then proceed to drive the parcours ahead of the riders, intermittently waving to the fans as they think I might be someone important. Obviously, this amuses me each and every time. It does break up the tedium, though, as you can be slouched in a car for up to six hours. In the car, I'll conduct more interviews. We usually bypass the finish line for the team hotel, where I'll interview the riders again, sometimes when they're having a massage. I've seen too many cyclists draped in only a towel the size of a flannel. I then eat more, enjoy a few pints chatting to whoever will listen (often no one) and hit bed at around 9 p.m. In short, eating, speaking, listening and driving. As for Rotunno...

- Early morning wake-up call and hopefully squeeze in a run.
- **6.30 a.m.** Visited by UCI anti-doping testers, who'll test the riders two or three times a week.
- **7.30 a.m.** Shovel breakfast down.

- **8 a.m.** Urine analysis of the riders and pre-breakfast weight check.
- **9 a.m.** Morning 'ward round' and dressing changes. This is to check the riders are healthy, and to clean and dress wounds.
- **10 a.m.** Pack up hotel room, hop on to bus and drive to starting village.
- **11.30 a.m.** Arrive at stage start. Team technical meeting to decide the day's tactics and the key players of the day. Then do a second weight check of the day to ensure hydration levels are fine. If not, advise further drinks containing electrolytes.
- **12.30 p.m.** Riders begin stage. I'll hit a team car or the bus and head to the finish with hopefully little activity between.
- **5 p.m.** Stage finish – hopefully a podium and anti-doping control thereafter.
- **5.15 p.m.** Find the bus! Then a quick rider check-up including a post-stage weigh-in for hydration levels, followed by transfer to the hotel, which is anywhere from 15km to 400km away.
- **7.30 p.m.** Evening 'ward round' to check riders are OK.
- **8.30 p.m.** Pharmacy run. This is to find the nearest open chemist – Google Maps is good here – to stock up on supplies.
- **9 p.m.** Another management tactical meeting.
- **9.30 p.m.** Dinner.
- **10.30 p.m.** Last-minute 'ward round'.
- **11.30 p.m.** Bed followed by tossing and turning in a room lacking air-conditioning!

It's an exhausting schedule during which Rotunno drains himself in the name of peak rider performance. His role is helped by state-of-the-art equipment but he's clear that one of the biggest things all of us can do, pro or otherwise, is neutralise the threat of infection by sanitising the environment.

'Hand gel was ubiquitous in the team even before Covid,' he says. 'We also insist that riders fist bump their fans. I'd actually prefer an elbow bump but that might be a little weird! Hygiene is critical. We are fastidious about hygiene.'

As are Ineos Grenadiers, who carved a reputation for cleanliness being next to godliness when it came to racing. (As it transpired, cleanliness might not have been next to godliness. Ineos' former, and banned, doctor, Richard Freeman, wrote in his book *The Line: Where Medicine and Sport Collide*[18], 'If there's infection in the toilet, which is highly likely, and you flush it with the lid open, you create an aerosol effect, so even if you've exited the bathroom or cubicle by the time that happens, you risk getting it on your toothbrush, so the next time you brush your teeth, you can pick up an infection.' I've been ensuring the lid is down ever since.)

At the end of the 2022 season, the British team had 12 medical staff on their books. On top of that, there were 12 carers plus three chefs and a nutritionist to ensure they were primed. Rotunno is part of a sizeable backroom team, too. Their job is to ensure the riders peak at their jobs. Rapid recovery equals more speed. Which is wonderful for the professionals. But what if you don't have Rotunno to check your hydration levels? Or Freeman to close the lid of your toilet seat? Just how achievable, and affordable, is rapid recovery when riding's not your job but squeezed in-between your job, family and social life?

'One of the things Whoop has opened my eyes to is that often the guys adapting to a multi-stage race are the ones sleeping well. Too many end up watching a film, reading, scrolling through social media … and they'll enjoy about six and a half hours sleep. Those who go straight to sleep enjoy eight or nine. That's effectively a day's more rest over the span of a Grand Tour, which is a huge benefit to performance.' These are the final words of EF doctor Kevin Sprouse before he leaves the meeting.

His remarks are certainly supported by anecdotal evidence. Years ago, I spent a working weekend with then Team Sky at the spring classic openers in Belgium at the tail end of February. On the Saturday is Omloop Het Nieuwsblad. One day later, around many of the same roads, is Kuurne–Brussels–Kuurne. It's a riotous two-day ride that not only kick-starts Flanders' season of hardcore, rugged professional cycling, but also sets in stone an official two-month doctrine from the Flandrean government that if you're caught without a Trappist beer in one hand, rolled-up race programme in the other and a head adorned with an upturned-peak cycling cap, you'll be exiled to the Ardennes.

Team Sky had made Hotel Messeyne in Kortrijk their base for many years and I got chatting to Luke Rowe about the stresses and strains of the Belgian double-header and whether or not it affected beauty kip. 'No, it's OK this weekend as it's relatively stress-free,' he replied with his Welsh lilt. 'But it's a different ballgame at the Tour de France. The heat, the media, the transfers... It's not overstating it to say that he who sleeps best often wins.'

These were the days when the British team dominated *La Grande Boucle* ('The Big Loop', aka the Tour de France) primarily through Chris Froome. The three-time winner had learned to lead a double life, morphing from a super-charged animal on his bike into a sloth off it. But only after trial and error that nearly burned him out. 'I once convinced myself that training once a day was stupid, so for a week all I did was train, sleep, eat, sleep, train, eat, sleep and ignored things like downtime and so on,' he wrote in *Shortlist* magazine[19]. 'I'd get back at 2 p.m., eat, sleep, then wake up at 8 p.m. and go out for another six-hour ride, then repeat the cycle. I was riding all through the night and sleeping during daylight, like a vampire who ignored the world around him. I only lasted four days. It wasn't healthy.'

Team Sky's sleep practices, including employing folk to carry the riders' portable air-conditioning units and other sleep accoutrements between hotels, made headlines as part of the theory of marginal gains. Froome is now with Israel–Premier Tech but still rides, and sleeps, within a team who place great importance on what you do between training and racing as well as during.

'Good sleep is without doubt the most fundamental aspects of effective recovery,' says Dr Ciarán O'Grady, performance coach at the Israel team. 'We work with Italian company Manifattura Falomo, who provide quality mattresses and pillows, in order to ensure that riders sleep on consistent surfaces every time they move hotels. It's not easy to ensure that beds at race hotels are good quality, so making sure the riders are sleeping comfortably and effectively is a big boost for their recovery.'

Seen through a performance lens, if I fail to sleep well, studies show that I'll suffer from decreased speed and power output, reduced reaction times, inhibited cognitive ability and an impaired immune system. In other words, I'll ride slower, crash because I'm an idiot and then take forever to heal. Which my wife would argue is me already, citing numerous examples, including the time I rode straight into a mesh metal fence at the bottom of a hill at the end of our road because I'd forgotten to connect my old-style brake callipers when attaching the front wheel. My descent of self-inflicted doom coincided with a mum, dad and toddler parking up and exiting their car to be greeted by Mr Bean flying past before crumpling like a sack of rather stupid spuds. 'I'm all good,' I'd assured them through the spokes as I lay on the tarmac. 'Just forgot to connect the brakes.' The family moved away soon after.

Off the bike, insufficient sleep can lead to weight gain, erratic mood, poor balance, memory issues and myriad heart conditions. Aside from the heart problems, again, I can relate to the other symptoms, especially the memory issues. Aside from the heart problems, again, I can relate to the other symptoms, especially the memory issues. . .

According to the NHS, the average Brit enjoys just six and a half hours' sleep a night with over a third at just five to six hours. The advent of smartphones – not that smart when it comes to sleep – social media, emails and instant messaging has rapidly eaten into sleep time. For me, it wasn't the advent of iPhones that signalled a sleep hit but our children. Now 23 and 18, the days of being woken at 3 a.m. for food or after some toilet incident are behind us, apart from when my son hits Bristol's clubs. However, those years of broken sleep seemingly shifted my body clock forever. Nowadays, it's rare that I wake after 6 a.m., usually more like 5 a.m. Yes, we hit the sack around 10 p.m. but I often wake for the loo, followed by a couple of hours struggling to sleep again, so I'm probably in that six-hour category at best. I wake early, drink coffee, drink another coffee, shower and then work.

With the training plan cranking up – the Sunday rides are growing in length each week and the Cheddar Gorge round trip is becoming commonplace, while I continue to spend most of the week training indoors – thoughts of boosting sleep to ease my passage up Alpe d'Huez seem fanciful. Things have improved slightly in recent times because my wife has invested in a new bed complete with topper, and critically, it lacks the foot railings of our previous bed, which had been fine for those under 1.8m – my wife – but not for those over – me. I'd learned the art of sleeping with my knees at a 60-degree kink to fit in it but clearly not mastered it as I'd still woken up often.

So, phones now banished from the bedroom. A bed that's actually long enough for me to stretch out in. Temperature at 17–18°C. Sheets instead of a thick duvet. Room darker than Lance's soul. Consistent bedtime. I'd ticked off the A–Z of good sleep etiquette but would still wake up feeling I lacked what I felt I needed. 'Maybe it's the alcohol and caffeine intake,' my wife suggested. That's where I played the sleep-deprived memory card, as well as burying my head deeply into the sands of ignorance. But I knew each played a part.

I'm not a daily drinker like many my age but I do enjoy a craft ale, of which Bristol offers numerous delightful options. New Bristol Brewery, Arbor, Wiper and True, Fierce and Noble ... if you're looking for an independent can of something hoppy that'll leave little change from a fiver, Bristol's your place. Friday and Saturday nights are definite drinking nights, with a quartet of pints on each. A Wednesday evening drink often breaks up the week. As for caffeine, I've always had at least three cups by 9 a.m. By lunchtime, that can hit five.

According to the Sleep Foundation, high amounts of alcohol cut sleep quality by 39.2 per cent. I'd argue the bar for 'high' rating is low at more than two drinks, which suggests I am in the high category, but the science says otherwise. They conclude that 'drinking alcohol before bed can add to the suppression of REM sleep during the first two cycles. Since alcohol is a sedative, sleep onset is often shorter for drinkers and some fall into deep sleep rather quickly. As the night progresses, this can create an imbalance between slow-wave sleep and REM [rapid eye movement] sleep, resulting in less of the latter and more of the former. This decreases overall sleep quality, which can result in shorter sleep duration and more sleep disruptions'.

Psychologically this is bad. Physiologically, it's not great, either, as sleep is when I'll rebuild and repair from the increase in training. A deeper dive into this impairment reveals it's all down to human growth hormone (HGH). The synthetic version was a staple of Lance Armstrong and his '90s ravers' medical cabinets. But for us innocent souls it's released in plentiful quantities from the brain's pituitary gland during both sleep and hard exercise. HGH repairs and rebuilds muscles by stimulating the liver and other tissues to make a protein called insulin-like growth factor 1 (IGF-1). Lack of sleep equals lack of HGH production equals restricted muscle growth. In fact, alcohol's a double blind-sider, not only impacting sleep but also decreasing secretion by 25 per cent.

As we all know, alcohol's the devil on the shoulder when it comes to food choices, as is lack of sleep. I already know the theory (but tend to try and forget I do): that it's all down to sleep shortage cranking up levels of a hormone called ghrelin. This signals that it's time to start eating. A German study[20] showed that just one night's broken sleep significantly raises ghrelin levels, explaining why you crave a tube of Pringles or unhealthy carb stodge when you're tired. The study also showed that two nights or more of poor sleep reduces the hormone leptin, which also regulates appetite.

It's no good. I'm going to have to go teetotal. Well, for a period anyway. If it doesn't help sleep, at least it'll cut some calories. And it really does. I lose weight through abstaining for a month and come to appreciate the flavours of Clear Head from the Bristol Beer Factory. It's alcohol-free but you can't tell, as it's rather delicious.

Of course, I've made that abstinence sound far easier than it was. Like many folk my age, there's a drinking pattern to the working week. With me, Monday night is football, so no drink; Tuesday is no drink as still feels too early; Wednesday? Hmm, midweek and all that. But my wife and I try to refrain. 'But a glass of wine won't do any harm,'

I speculate. Usually on a weekly basis. So, in theory, Wednesday is a no; in practice, it's often a go. Thursday depends on how stressful the day's been. So, usually, a glass or two. Friday and Saturday is carte blanche. Sunday for me is no. For my wife, a yes. Which means often a yes from me. This is a long-winded way of saying I found it much harder to abstain from alcohol than I did hopping on to an indoor trainer first thing in the morning!

But did cutting booze help me kip? Well, it certainly helped reduce nocturnal urine visits. But it wasn't perfect. I suspect cortisol's the bigger problem for me. A particularly stressful year (bike break-in, house sale, wife's long Covid, son's A-level exams, struggling to find a new house to buy, work...) has not left me cradling the Dalai Lama in a gong bath while my resting heart rate matches that of Miguel Induráin (a reported 27bpm at his 1990s' pomp). Much is made in the world today of turning everything into a positive. That it's stress that gets you out of bed. That it drives you to break down barriers. I agree. To a point. Cross that point, as I did in much of 2022, and it manifests in perma-fatigue and, strangely, aching legs. Whenever I'm highly stressed, my legs ache, much more so than they do from cycling and football. It's the oddest thing, though several studies place the blame on raised cortisol levels, which over time deplete your adrenal glands. Apparently, this raises the body's sensitivity to pain. I am a delicate flower.

Or are the sleep-broken nights down to exercise late in the day? As I mentioned at the start of this journey, five-a-side brings huge joy – alongside a huge dollop of adrenaline. That certainly disrupts Monday-night shut-eye but that's the only real time I exercise past 7 p.m. so I'm not sure it explains my problems during the rest of the week.

All that said, I'm not an insomniac, so at least I know I'm getting a fair amount of sleep. But even so, I once again contact Israel team doctor O'Grady to tap him for any other recovery tips I can steal from the pros. 'Between each stage the riders will all have a massage. These practitioners may use ultrasound therapy to aid recovery, as well as SpiderTech taping. The riders also have access to the Hyperice

Normatec boots, which provide pulsing compression to the riders' legs, allowing them to start their recovery in the bus on the way to the hotel after the stage. Riders might also use the Hyperice Hypervolt, a mobile massage gun, to prepare their legs ready for the massage treatment at the hotel.

'The vast majority of riders find a benefit in the massage process,' the soothing O'Grady continues. 'Some simply find it beneficial to have a quiet place to relax and switch off after a hectic stage. The masseur usually has a very close relationship with riders, so the sharing of family news or discussing of other personal topics is quite common, so the massage treatment can be more than just a physical recovery tool. From a physical perspective, the massage helps the rider's body to relax and boost the recovery process. There is also the ability to detect any potential musculoskeletal issues before they become problems, such as tight muscles or imbalances.'

Armed with this knowledge, I sign up to a sports massage on our local high street. Yet another expense. Inflation's flying. Can I justify a rub-down? As it transpired, the massage was fine but not fine enough to warrant becoming another monthly direct debit. The frugal father in me says leave it unless you really need it. So, I give compression socks a go. Or, as some wag nicknamed them, 'contraception socks'. They're the affordable version of high-tech boots like the Hyperice Normatec and resemble football socks, albeit ones that are three sizes too small. Their mooted benefits derive from near-tourniquet levels of pressure and sexy they are not. Every WorldTour training camp I've ever attended resembles a Lowry painting; the limbs of these cycling matchstick men sketched even leaner because of the contraception socks they all wander around in.

They're certainly function over form, the idea being that every time you move, your calf squeezes the veins of the lower limb to send blood back to the heart to offload the carbon dioxide and onboard more oxygen. Compression wear gives this process a helping hand, which is why fit is so important. Compression is measured in millimetres of mercury (mmHg), which is a unit of pressure and more commonly applied to blood pressure. A normal resting blood pressure is 120/80mmHg. The top figure (systolic) is blood pressure in your arteries when your heart beats; the bottom figure (diastolic) is blood pressure in your arteries when your heart rests between beats.

'That blood pressure obviously lowers [in regions of the body that are further] away from the heart and is why many compression manufacturers settle on around 22mmHg at the ankle and 18mmHg at the thigh, but these values vary between manufacturers,' reads a British Association of Sport and Exercise Sciences (BASES) official statement on compression. Sizing is vital and manufacturers feature a wide range of options.

The theory stands up but do they work in practice? Studies are equivocal and many point the finger at the placebo effect, the theory being that the cradling of the limbs tells your brain this has benefits, which then perks up your mood, which in turn delivers a physical boost. As for me, I spend a few weeks cycling and walking around in a pair of socks from Compressport that I'd dug out of my sports drawer from years past. Did they work? They were certainly performance-enhancing to squeeze into, prepping my triceps muscles for the bar-pulling strain of Alpe d'Huez and raising my metabolism. Once on, they felt comfortable enough but the aches persisted. Was I using them in the incorrect physical situation? Probably. But when I'd used them in the past, it had been post-run. As I've banged on about with my Monday-night footy, the muscle tears and micro-damage of running are far greater than weight-bearing cycling. Despite professional cyclists using them, at a recreational level I'd argue they're better for runners than cyclists.

Ultimately, coach Mosley's training plan for me provided one of the best forms of recovery. 'Avoid back-to-back hard sessions,' he ordered. 'And include at least one rest day in the week, plus include an active recovery week every fourth week. They're about half the training you do in a normal week. They're good not just because it helps you recovery physically, but it's a mental break as well. People often spend a little more time with their families.'

This works wonders for the mind. In general, I'm riding four times a week plus the kickabout. There's commuting thrown into that mix, too. The midweek rides are fine – they're rarely over 90 minutes and include one easier ride. It's the weekly longer ride that can chafe as it just takes up so much time. This recovery training balm every four weeks becomes vital.

After playing around with myriad recovery ideas and tools, I'm still not sleeping wonderfully and suspect that ultimately this is down to my internal body clock. This is the clock deep within the brain, which regulates internal systems such as eating and sleeping patterns. Our body clock also regulates temperature, alertness, mood and digestion in a 24-hour process evolved to work in harmony with the Earth's rotation. Our body clocks are set by external cues, chief among them being daylight. Recent advances have revealed that the functioning of our bodies is affected far more extensively by circadian rhythm than was previously known. We now know that one out of every 10 genes in human DNA operates in a 24-hour cycle.

'There's increasing scientific evidence to support the informal concept of "owls" and "larks"', explains Professor David Bishop, senior sports scientist at Victoria University in Australia and an authority on the subject. 'It's because most of our bodily processes vary over an approximate 24-hour cycle, meaning we have mental and physical peaks and troughs.

'There's no doubt that cycling performance changes throughout the day,' continues Bishop. 'In our own studies, we've shown that maximal sprint power is greater in the afternoon. This coincides with peak of body temperature, which increases factors such as nerve conduction velocity, flexibility and blood flow. Endurance performance seems to be less affected by time of day than power, although we've reported better endurance performance in the evening compared to the morning.'

Despite this broad brush, circadian rhythms don't strictly adhere to the 24-hour clock; in fact, they vary slightly by individual with about an hour's range from 23.8 hours to 24.8 hours. This 'slow' or 'fast' clock relates to evening or morning types with reportedly 10 per cent qualifying as morning people, 20 per cent night owls and the rest in the large spectrum in-between. That time shift doesn't sound huge but it has significant repercussions, with one study showing evening types can see performance levels drop by as much as 26 per cent when training in the morning compared to the evening. It's why some suggest morning larks peak around noon, in-betweeners around 4 p.m. and night owls around 8 p.m.

So, it seems that chronotype (your body's circadian rhythm) may be important to peak cycling performance. More important than a liking for the finest craft ale and super-strong coffee, I hope. Fantastic. This is out of my hands; in fact, I'll point the finger at my mother and father. Actually, probably my mum. My dad's borderline narcoleptic, his favourite recliner casting a soporific spell over him every time he sits down. Mum's the opposite, seeing broken sleep as the norm.

I've always preferred morning exercise and the majority of my rides in preparation for the Étape are in the morning. Later on, after the mental rather than physical exertions of the day, I feel fatigued. My brain's already endured a day's workload and as that's the control centre that dictates tiredness, perceptively if not physically, I feel tired. That's my feeling, anyway. But what does the science say? That's when I come across the awkwardly titled Morningness-Eveningness questionnaire[21], an online assessment of whether you're a lark or an owl or in-between.

Example questions include: 'You have decided to do physical exercise. A friend suggests that you do this for one hour twice a week, and the best time for him is 7–8am. How do you think you would perform?' You have a choice of four answers. Mine? 'Would be in good form,' thank you very much.

'If you got into bed at 11pm, how tired would you be?' 'Very tired.' In fact, crawling up the walls. Life at 45 years old is indeed rock and roll.

My score is 78, which is slap bang in the middle of the 'definite morning' category. So, I'm training to my internal body clock optimum. That's good. This could explain why I rise early. That's good. My start time for L'Étape du Tour is 7.52 a.m. That's good. The finish time could be anywhere up to midnight! That's bad. I'd better get my shrinking arse in gear and aim to finish around the time of the 2019 winner Adrien Guillonnet, who completed the last (pre-Covid) amateur Tour stage in 4.44.11. Do that and I'll be done by lunchtime, making my chronotype very happy indeed.

8

Fuelling Dreams

T-minus two months

Witham Friary is a sleepy English village between the eclectic town of Frome and the small town of Bruton. The heart of this Somerset idyll is St Mary's Church, a Grade I listed building that dates back to the 1200s (though it is built on the site of a seventh-century church). On this summer's eve, bunting flutters in the warm breeze, nettles gently protect farmhouse after farmhouse, and magnificent oaks take easy centre stage in rolling fields. It's an incongruous, though perhaps much-needed, backdrop for a Londoner whose role is one of the most frenetic and most important in modern-day professional road riding: the team chef.

'Welcome to Holt Farm,' Owen Blandy, team chef at EF Education–EasyPost, says as he greets me at the door of his farmhouse, dressed in casual grey T-shirt, blue football shorts, flip-flops and brown cap, from which a curl of black fringe pokes out. 'Coffee?'

Blandy is 35. He grew up in London, dreamed of becoming a professional footballer, has a background in chartered accountancy, ran his own fixed-gear bike team that competed around the world in the uber-cool Red Hook Criterium series ... and has somehow ended up in a village right out of the *Midsomer Murders*. At least, that is, when he's not cooking for the likes of Magnus Cort Nielsen and Rigoberto Urán in the pressure-cooker environs of the Tour de France.

Back at the farmhouse, I reply in the affirmative to the offer of coffee. 'I won't have one as I've been living on a litre of the stuff a day for the past month. I covered the whole Giro and will do the Tour and Vuelta. That'll be six Grand Tours in a row. You know Adam Hansen?'

I nod. I've interviewed the retired Australian domestique before, most recently in his new guise as an Ironman triathlete. 'Well, I'm chasing his record of 20 Grand Tours in succession.' Blandy smiles, while meticulously measuring out coffee beans from Girona for one Americano with a dash of milk and one sugar.

I've driven the hour and a quarter from Bristol to understand the demands and needs of cyclists who often burn through 8000 calories a day, possess body-fat levels that reach as low as 5 per cent and are often type-A personalities whose standards are consistently, almost brutally, high. I'll also look for some easy nutritional advice to take home.

I've interviewed many team chefs in their professional domain before, including Ineos Grenadiers' Jon Cox in Antwerp and Trek–Segafredo's Kim Rokkjaer in Pau. But that was in the racing amphitheatre, where time is as limited as patience. Now, with a small break between Grand Tours, a relaxed Blandy has invited me into his life away from cycling ... to talk cycling.

But before we mull over macronutrients, discover the secret to the perfect cyclist's omelette and talk rice cakes, I'm keen to find out how Blandy joined the tight community of WorldTour chefs.

'It's a bit of a strange one... Sorry, let me just put the sourdough in.' Blandy lifts a tea towel off a dough-filled bread tin, and places it in what looks like an oversized black reception bell. 'That's an iron cloche. It creates an oven within an oven. Bakeries will have steam-injected ovens, which gives the sourdough a really nice crust and that chewy sourdough flavour that you buy for five quid a loaf. This replicates it. I do this for the riders and bake sourdough for them every day of a Grand Tour. JV [Jonathan Vaughters, the charismatic manager of Blandy's team] loves my sourdough pancakes.'

I've attempted to bake sourdough before. It didn't go well. 'All I know about sourdough is that people can become obsessed by their sourdough starters [the frothy mixture of wild yeast, flour and water that is used to leaven the bread in place of commercial yeast or a raising agent such as bicarbonate of soda],' I say. 'Yep, that's me. Mine's 12 years old. It's why I'll always leave some here when I'm on the road in case it's lost. JV suggests it should be transported around on Air Force One. Right, where were we? Ahh yes, how I ended up here…

'Well, I grew up in London and loved sport. I played football, trained with the Arsenal FC Academy but didn't make it. I studied sports science at Leeds University but ended up back in London working for a property company. They had an asset management department and I started doing cashflow for them. I stayed for six or seven years. Went to Rothschild in investment management at St James Place. And then started my chartered accountancy qualification.

'But I always had a passion for food, so for a year I combined my day job with stints at a gastro-pub in Chiswick and Hawksmoor [a steak restaurant] in London. But it wasn't the cooking I wanted to do; I didn't want to be hidden out back or in a basement and not connect with the end user of the food. So, I gave up on "cheffing", finished my qualification – after four years and 14 exams – though I soon realised [that having the charted accountancy qualification would only be useful as] only as a back-up. I just wanted to cook. Then the pandemic struck and I decided I wanted out of London pretty early on. That's when I called Seth…'

Seth Tabatznik was an old school friend of Blandy's in London. In 2015, Seth and his sister, Lara, conceived the idea of a retreat with sustainability at its core. They searched around, discovered the land right next to where Blandy would move to – the farmhouse in Witham Friary – and founded 42 Acres. The idea is that people can reconnect with nature and by doing so reconnect with themselves. It's a magnificent space, featuring a lake to wild swim. 42 Acres also has two polytunnels, a walled garden, and follows organic and permaculture principles, from which skilled chefs cook for the guests.

'I'm really interested in the source of food and told Seth I wanted to come and work for him. That was my doorway back into cooking.'

That was 2020. Later in the year, Blandy got chatting with another old friend, Will Girling. Girling's the long-time nutritionist of EF. Their paths had crossed when Girling sought high-level amateur athletes for his PhD looking at carbohydrate utilisation. Blandy, a keen cyclist, was one of the subjects he tested in the performance department at Saracens rugby training ground and they've remained friends ever since. 'Will mentioned they were looking for a chef. I'd never worked in cycling but applied. The next minute I'm at Paris–Nice, cooking on my own for the world's best cyclists. It was nerve-wracking but it helped being a cyclist. I know what you want to eat. And I kept it simple – functional eating for sports performance. After that first month, they said I'd done well and that was it.'

When the riders briefly hibernate, Blandy returns to 42 Acres to cook and learn more about the perma-principles of this hypnotically tranquil backdrop. But when the clocks spring forwards and the sun strengthens, Blandy shifts up a gear or 11 and hits the road.

'I'd better check that bread,' Blandy interrupts, making a beeline for the oven within the oven. 'You want it as hot as possible for around 25 minutes. You then turn it down, remove the lid and bake for another 20 minutes.'

We head from the magnificent farmhouse kitchen to the garden. There's a pear tree, an apple tree, chillies hanging out to dry and herbs everywhere. 'You've done well for yourself,' I comment. 'This isn't mine, sadly,' Blandy says. 'I rent it with two couples from a lady opposite who's a retired doctor. She's interested in micro-farming and Hannah, one of my housemates, looks after around 50 cows. They're the happiest cows in the land and are 100 per cent pasture fed. We'll eat one later.'

So not that happy. Unlike me, since I've just spotted two of the most appetising-looking steaks I've ever seen resting on the side.

'Do the riders eat much red meat,' I ask Blandy? 'They'd like to but when we're at Grand Tours, we'll only cook it for them the night before a rest day. It just sits in the stomach too long digesting during the race itself. JV is a great believer in red meat and says it's good for red blood cells. Maybe it is but it's just extra weight. Still, I did pack a load of the meat, including tomahawks and fillet steaks, in my suitcase and cook a barbecue for riders and staff several days before a Grand Tour. They loved it – until I posted a picture of the cow it came from on WhatsApp.'

JV raced in the 1990s, when arguably the prevalence of doping meant that nutrition was an afterthought. Now, in hopefully cleaner times, nearly every team has its own nutritionist and chef. Sports nutrition scientist Asker Jeukendrup, whom we came across in Chapter 4, charted this fuelling evolution in a webinar he hosted via his Mysportscience online platform during the 2022 Tour de France. Jeukendrup's many roles include heading up nutrition at Jumbo–Visma, and during the webinar he explained how the Dutch team's fuelling strategy has changed over the years.

'In 2017, we started working with a company who would deliver us pre-prepared healthy meals [that] we'd heat up. In 2018, I worked directly with two riders and tried to make things more targeted, so amounts and macronutrients specific to that particular rider. It was an enormous amount of work and not scalable. Thankfully, in 2019, the team launched an app that replaced my spreadsheet. We weighed foods so knew exactly what the riders were consuming. The team also invested in a food truck, and the number of chefs and nutritionists grew to six. That rose to nine in 2020 and 11 in 2021 for both the men's and women's teams.'

Jumbo–Visma has arguably overtaken Ineos Grenadiers as the most progressive team on the WorldTour, certainly in the culinary stakes. That's down to an increasing budget and working with one of their sponsors, supermarket chain Jumbo, which affords an individualisation that's impressive.

'Planning for the Tour de France starts months in advance,' says Jeukendrup. 'We know what the parcours is and can make a plan for each stage. We then make a series of nutritional predictions for each stage. These are based on who's going to ride the Tour and the physiology of each rider. For each stage and the potential role and goal of each rider, we can then predict their power output and intensity of effort, and so can predict energy expenditure and carbohydrate use. This'll involve many members of staff: the directeurs sportifs, coaches, riders, performance nutritionist, head of nutrition… This is where meal planning and the team chefs come in. With this information, they can start to formulate meals for each stage. The Jumbo Food Coach app plays an important role here as it tells the athlete what to eat and monitors what they eat.'

This is the preparation. The application, Jeukendrup continues, can be tinkered with as soon as the stage is over. 'When the riders stop their power meters, all the data from there, including power output and calories burnt, is sent to the Cloud. The chefs can now work with live data and adapt their meal plans if necessary.'

It's impressively precise, detailed stuff that, as Jeukendrup says, is all about the delivery and adaptability. Which Jumbo–Visma did with metronomic consistency at the 2022 Tour de France, of course, resulting in Jonas Vingegaard winning the yellow jersey plus six stage wins for the team including three from Wout van Aert.

'Today was the perfect day to highlight how the actual result changes the nutritional prediction,' adds performance nutritionist Martijn Redegeld, picking up the fuelling baton from Jeukendrup in the same webinar[22]. 'Wout was in the break for most of the day [stage six] and rode the last part solo. We based our calculations on him being in the break but could see he was on form so increased his predicted power output, which meant a greater carbohydrate intake. Once he'd crossed the line, we were still below his actual power output, so upped the carbohydrate intake again. He'll be having a lot of chicken nuggets tonight!' Redegeld references team chef Karen Lambrechtse, who announced that she was cooking the riders healthy and homemade nuggets that evening, along with fresh bread, vegetables and homemade/squeezed juice.

EF Education–EasyPost has one of the smaller budgets. It means Blandy is currently the sole chef but, by working in unison with Girling, he still achieves the Grand Tour aim of helping each and every rider reach the finish line at around the weight at which they started the race.

Maintaining race weight is a sign that the body is avoiding a catabolic state whereby it enters starvation mode and begins burning higher quantities of protein as fuel, often in the form of muscle. If the body starts cannibalising itself, power drops, fatigue sets in and you have a rider who's often on the verge of illness and withdrawal.

This fact means that there must have been a peloton of malnourished athletes cycling around in France in 1911 at the ninth edition of the Tour. A study Jeukendrup presented showed that, on average, riders lost 7.1 per cent of their bodyweight over the 5343km 15-stage race that started in Paris with a 351km romp to Dunkirk on stage one and finished back in Paris 14 stages later after a final 317km trawl from Le Havre. The greatest loss was suffered by Belgian Louis Heusghem, whose weight plummeted from 83kg to 73.5kg. If those figures were seen in the 21st century, the fuelling team would be shown the (oven) door.

Back at Holt Farm, Blandy has removed the loaf of sourdough from the oven. It looks and smells like it has been baked by the gods. By serving this heavenly morsel to the riders each day, rich in yeasty goodness, he says, their gut biome and health are emboldened, which is needed come the third and final week of a Grand Tour when their digestive systems are doing cartwheels. That's despite a diet that's almost devoid of fibre.

'In a race, that insoluble fibre in the gut is just dead weight,' says Blandy. 'It can also irritate the stomach when working hard. It's why we limit fibre to less than 10g a day and is why when it comes to breakfast, I'll always put out Corn Flakes and Rice Krispies. Those cereals are high in sugar and low in fibre, so exactly what they need.

'I'll also peel every vegetable I cook, to remove the fibrous skin, and it's why we rarely have broccoli and kale,' Blandy continues. 'In fact, Alberto Bettiol [who won the Tour of Flanders in 2019] doesn't have any fibre at all and barely touches vegetables, as he has Crohn's disease. It can set off an autoimmune response so, for him, it's really about pasta, rice, meat and fish, though I will do cold-pressed juice for him and remove all the fibre.'

With 31 riders from 20 nationalities to cook for – albeit not all at the same time – I ask Blandy about catering for specific rider needs among a large group of athletes of different ages and different background. He says, as a whole, the group are pretty easy but he and Girling keep a spreadsheet of the riders' tolerances and allergies, tapping into his accountancy past. 'There are no coeliacs, which is unusual, but we have a couple of vegetarians: Owain Doull and Jonas Rutsch. They're interesting to cook for and enjoy foods like tofu and seitan, but they do need to take extra protein shakes and bars as it's hard to consume as many vegetable calories as meat calories. Around 100g of steak contains 30g protein; 100g tofu's half that. Thankfully, they eat eggs as not only does this provide good calories and protein, but it's a breakfast staple.'

Which brings us to Blandy's daily culinary tour at the Tour, where eggs, which are good for muscle repair and nerve function, dominate. 'I have a food truck where I store and cook a lot of my food but, when it comes to breakfast, I'll cook omelettes for the riders every morning over an induction hob that I'll take into the hotel's dining room.' I tapped him up for his perfect omelette recipe.

'I'll use spray as it disperses the oil evenly over the pan and use olive or avocado oil. I'll then whip the eggs until fluffy, which takes a couple of minutes. I saw someone on YouTube do it in a blender and it was almost like a souffle it had that much air in it. But a fork is fine.

'Keep the pan at six out of 10 heat and take it off when it's cooking too much. Once you see a skin of egg, you can roll it around the pan from one side to the other and just keep cooking slowly. When it's cooked, ideally it should be pure yellow with no browning; it should be like a pillow on the outside and a scrambled-egg finish on the inside but some like it cooked more. If adding a filling, don't go overboard. A tablespoon of grated cheese and half a slice of ham is fine. Any more and you might split the egg.'

Blandy is an egg enthusiast and knows his team's requirements inside out, apart from one. 'Hugh Carthy will have a massive plate of rice – all the riders have rice for breakfast, jasmine or Thai as it's more flavoursome – with an omelette beside but he'll play games with me.

He'll say, "Two", meaning two eggs and two whites. Or "Three one", meaning three eggs and one white. He confessed he had no idea what he was talking about, he was just amusing himself.

'Some riders have the same omelette every morning. It's like clockwork. Magnus [Cort] has two eggs, ham and cheese. Rigo [Urán] has three eggs, ham, cheese and no pepper. I've noticed that the most successful riders keep it simple. They rarely ask for anything different on the food table; they don't waste energy on things they don't have to. They'll be the last down to the hotel foyer [before a stage start] with their bags and I'm sure they're just as efficient at energy saving in the peloton.'

This efficiency spreads through the team. Chefs will aim to feed the riders around three hours before the stage start, though occasionally they'll have a smaller Tupperware container of rice and eggs for the morning transfer. And similar, maybe with some veg, for the hotel transfer from the stage finish later in the day.

In the meantime, while the riders ride, Blandy drives his food truck to the next hotel and preps for dinner. 'The truck's packed with good-quality, organic essentials like tinned tomatoes, but for something like the Giro and Tour, you'll have a food budget from the organisers. I'll then drop the hotel we're staying at after each stage an email and their staff will source the extra food (fish, chicken, vegetables...) for my recipes. ASO [Amaury Sport Organisation, who organise the Tour] even provide a menu for the smaller teams who don't have a chef and the hotel team will cook it.

'I work a day ahead so the team are actually providing my ingredients for the next day,' Blandy continues. 'The last thing you want is to turn up to the hotel and [discover] the fish is crap. Most are great but I remember one kitchen at the Vuelta a España, which was so dirty I didn't accept any of the food.'

As Blandy starts on our dinner – rice (what else?), vegetables and home-slaughtered steak – I look for some culinary feedback on the respective Grand Tours. 'Practically, France is the easiest because the roads are best and transfers are good. And ASO is very good at organising. There's even a guy who's responsible for checking the quality of ingredients at hotels. He'll phone you up and say don't use the chicken, its best before is today. Italy's the most beautiful place we race and some of the hotels are amazing. As is how they present their food. But there can be long transfers and winding roads. It's the same with Spain. You forget how vast it is. There's a massive transfer at this year's Vuelta of around 900km from the Basque region to the south-east coast. I'll drive alone. It's quite tiring.'

Tiring but rewarding. Blandy's enthusiasm is high, this being just his second year. His love of the sport combined with a love of food, its provenance and the scientific application for cyclists makes this his dream job. And that drive and energy is needed as his race days are long, prepping for food as early as 6 a.m. and serving up dinner around 14 hours later. He's become smarter over the past couple of seasons, he says, using the hotels' cutlery and plates, for instance, as they'll be more likely to wash it for you.

'OK, the veg is ready.' Blandy has sliced and fried ginger, garlic, courgette and French beans, the latter duo grown locally. He's also removed the jasmine rice from the hob to finish steam cooking for the 10 minutes it takes to cook and rest the steak.

'I'll just slice off much of that fat as I like to use that to cook the steak in,' Blandy explains, before he sets to with the meat. 'It's a mix of Hereford and Shetland,' says housemate Laura who has joined us. 'For meat-eaters like me, it's the stuff of carnivorous dreams.'

'A lot of supermarket steaks are raised via bulk feeding, which produces big nodules of fat,' Blandy continues. 'If a cow's grazing on grass like here, the fat slowly intersperses into muscle. It means better marbling, better flavour and a healthier cow.'

The cows at Meadow Sweet are hung for three weeks and then customers have three weeks to order. Sadly, I'm not taking a cut but you can find out more at www.meadowsweetbeef.co.uk. It'll be worth your time and money as it's stunning, melting in the mouth and juicily delicious. The whole meal's simple but impressive, ticking many a nutritional box and not requiring much time to make or eat, all of which is important in the WorldTour kitchen.

It's time to leave Holt Farm. I head home, navigating the tight country lanes, reflecting on an intellectually and nutritionally rewarding evening. But then one regret floods over me. How could this have happened? Why, why, why? We forgot to eat the ambrosial sourdough.

———

'So, just need to make one thing clear, you don't want to forego your successful and rewarding career in teaching and become my "team" chef?' My efforts at turning my wife into the next Blandy fell on deaf, slightly aggressive ears. The same with my daughter and son. Disappointingly disloyal. But ne'er mind. I might lack the finances to pay for the application of textbook cycling nutrition but I can afford a customised theoretical session. In other words, an analysis of my current 'fuelling programme' by sports nutritionist Emily Kier.

Kier is a freelancer who often helps out leading sports dietitian Renee McGregor. I'd interviewed McGregor many moons ago but her name drifted from my orbit over time. That was until a late-February, late-18th-birthday visit to Lisbon with my son, Harold (Harry, but for some reason it amuses me to call him Harold. Which doesn't amuse my wife. Which amuses me even more). While we were there, Harold/Harry had kindly bought me a sightseeing tour of this historic Portuguese city. What a thoughtful gift, I thought. But I soon didn't think that when it became clear this was a running sightseeing tour at 7 a.m. on the first morning of our trip. 'Good training for the book,' he said with a grin. Hmm…

Anyway, he was right – it was good training for the book as the host, Pedro, turned out to be a former Ironman athlete who seemed incapable of jogging. Instead, it flowed into a high-intensity interval session that passed in a blur. On one brief recovery segment, Pedro explained to me how a British nutritionist had helped him secure a spot at the daddy of all Ironman events: Hawaii. 'This lady was a genius,' he said. 'She helped me lose weight and race better by encouraging me to eat more. Her name was Renee McGregor.'

Lose weight. Eat more. What modern-day witchcraft was this? Back in England, I dropped Renee an email, and she passed me on to the equally well-equipped Kier to see if she could work the same magic with me. You see, I've always been active and up until around the age of 32 or 33, the fatty deposits had remained relatively absent. Then, whether it was a move closer to Bristol meaning a shorter daily commute on the bike or simply my body slowing down, suddenly lipids decided to infiltrate my back and other, till then, leaner areas. Not a tsunami but a gradual drip-feeding that, over 10 years, saw my weight creep up from around 83kg to around 92kg, which is where it was at the start of this Étape training journey. I knew that I would drop a few pounds with the training – though greater weight loss was needed for me to do well in the mountains – but I'd entered the danger zone. I'm far from obese and am relatively fit but I am in the age group 45 to 74. According to the NHS, age-wise this is the obese group (albeit an all-encompassing one by range as well as waistline), which is down to myriad reasons, including muscle degradation, reduced physical activity and metabolic slowdown.

'One of the most striking effects of age is the involuntary loss of muscle mass, strength and function, termed sarcopenia,' say the authors of the 2004 paper 'Muscle Tissue Changes with Aging'[23]. The article continues, 'A decrease in muscle mass is also accompanied by a progressive increase in fat mass and consequently changes in body composition.' Not great visually or for long-term health. 'All these changes have probable implications for several conditions, including type-2 diabetes, obesity, heart disease and osteoporosis.'

All are highly undesirable and while the thought of climbing three Alpine mountains in one day, trampled on by temperatures that could kiss 50°C roadside, may be slightly scary, that's nothing compared to spending a good percentage of your life with a life-limiting condition. The long-term benefits of habitual exercise and good nutrition far outweigh any short-term discomfort.

'Send me over a week's normal food intake and meals and we'll take it from there,' Kier emailed. So, I did, telling the truth, the whole truth and nothing but the truth. Generally, as a family, we eat well. We look to cook fresh where possible and don't pack the cupboards with too many unhealthy snacks. I'm no snacker but I do like a packet of crisps. Not fancy, mind. I'll rarely deviate from ready salted or salt and vinegar. Anyway, here's a food-diary snapshot:

Breakfast: Homemade smoothie with frozen fruit, a spoonful of protein powder, crushed nuts and around 400ml milk.
AM snack: Packet of crisps.
Lunch: Chicken in pitta bread with salad and a packet of crisps.
PM snack: Muesli bar.
Dinner: Lasagne plus a slice of garlic bread and a green salad.
Pudding: N/A.
Drinks: Four to five cups of coffee with one sugar and semi-skimmed milk. Two to three bottles of water.
Alcohol: Three cans of 500ml ale (5%).
Supplements: Multivitamin, vitamin C, vitamin D, cod liver oil.

I leave my food diary with Kier and send over my blood reports from Chapter 4. I also tell her about my basal metabolic results from Chapter 1, which is just under 1900 calories, and email over my training plan of around six to nine hours' exercise a week plus football. I'm pretty good with the theory of sports nutrition and feel confident about working out my race nutrition, but how's my general diet in practice?

'Not bad,' says Kier. 'But we just need a few tweaks.' Let the tweaks begin...

'OK, let's start with breakfast. It looks like you generally ride early on just coffee, so fasted. Some studies say it's OK for men to train fasted...' I know this bit already – one study was carried out by Dr James Morton from Chapter 1, who recommended the technique of riding with low glycogen levels to boost fat burning and mitochondrial numbers for better performance to Team Sky. '...My personal opinion is that it's not needed for recreational athletes. It might be for a multi-stage race, especially if you're not supported like in the Marathon des Sables, but you might benefit more by even just having half a banana before.'

That's easily done. Kier also advises a slice of toast to accompany the smoothie for an extra carbohydrate hit. It'll replenish glycogen levels, which isn't just important for recovery but also to be relatively sharp for the working day ahead.

'We can work on that morning snack, too,' Kier continues. 'I don't mind the occasional packet of crisps but they're essentially air and oil. A handful of nuts, oatcakes with hummus, a slice of bread with cream cheese...' To be fair, often we'll have almonds to hand but generally only if we have got around to doing an online weekly shop. If that doesn't happen, if life gets in the way, goodness drops sharply alongside an increase in takeaways.

Lunch seems to tick most boxes though I should seek a good-fat source, too, like avocado or more nuts. 'You could have another chicken breast, though, to boost muscle-repairing protein. But your carbs don't look too bad. You're a writer so you have a sedentary job, so you don't need to go mad with those.' Too sedentary. It was only when I completed Kier's form that I realised just how much I sit down throughout the day: I work from 7–8 a.m. (or from 8 a.m. if not working from home and an early morning bike commute's required) through to 5–6 p.m. and spend most of that time sitting in front of a screen. It's an unhealthy way to live, especially now I'm in my mid-40s. There's the exercise, of course, though most of that's sitting down. Or walking, of course, when it comes to steep cobbles...

'Dinner looks OK but always aim for the five-finger rule,' Kier says. 'That's a carb source, protein, good fats and at least two vegetables. So, if you're having a salad, mix it up with leafage, tomatoes...

'Then again, you're not a professional rider who often has their meals cooked for them, certainly at training camp,' Kier continues. 'Sometimes you might just want pasta and pesto for lunch, which lacks protein. That's fine. Just remember later to have some nuts as a snack or chicken for dinner. Snacks are a great way to fill any macronutrient gaps you might have.'

During the analysis period, my family and I were giving Gousto a go. I'd been seduced by the big discounts over the first four weeks, so had signed up. We also tried Hello Fresh for a week but preferred Gousto. It had been a particularly busy year. The house sale was edging closer, meaning packing up 14 years of memories, books and rubbish. My wife's long Covid had put her out of action. Her predicament was far greater than mine but sharing tasks now became my tasks. And our kids who were no longer kids remained as domestically useless as I was at 18 and 23! So, beyond the savings, the idea of food and recipes being delivered to the door was tempting. It would also shake things up a little as cooking at home so much during Covid had drained the culinary imagination somewhat, especially as I've always been the cook. It proved a worthwhile exercise. Not only were the recipes easy and tasty – I'm not on commission – but they taught portion control. I've always thought my main problem is meal size, namely too big. This is exaggerated as I'm the main cook, so I tend to take the chef's mantra of you 'must taste and season' to the extreme. Often, by the time I serve up, I'm nearly full.

This Gousto trial only lasted a month, however. Despite the variety, size, taste and convenience, the evening meal began to lose its allure. With the delivery scheme, it was all too mechanical – understandably, everything was packaged, meaning our fridge resembled a warehouse. It's hardly eco-friendly, either. So, it was goodbye Gousto and a return to 'normal' cooking – spag bog, pasta and pesto, the occasional roast! – for this tired chef.

Kier and I also looked into fuelling evening sessions. Because of the flexibility of my job (writing can drain time but, in general, you can choose the time of day that it drains) and the fact I mostly ride solo, as I've mentioned I tend to train first thing. But once a week, football starts at 8 p.m. and finishes at 9.15 p.m., meaning that I don't eat until about 10. 'I'd cook dinner and have half before and half after,' says Kier, 'and make sure you let it digest for an hour. Better to have shorter, better-quality sleep than longer, broken sleep.' We talked about bulk cooking couscous, the genius of jacket potatoes and losing a few pounds through cutting alcohol, which I'd tried (*see* Chapter 7) and would do again in the month before the Étape.

Kier's input was useful and the changes were affordable. I was relieved to realise my diet didn't need an overhaul, just refining. Also, I'm not going to have to live like a monk. I duly begin to work on portion size. Thankfully, the teenage days of building a food mountain on my plate are well behind me...

And yet, one Friday lunchtime in May, I find myself at Toby Carvery, Middlemoor, Exeter – the city in which I grew up. The sun is shining, so I'm sitting on a bench outside enjoying some rays. Inside, the diligent staff are cleaning up from breakfast and prepping for lunch. Gone are the hash browns, fried eggs and Yorkshire pudding – yes, Toby serves up a breakfast Yorkie – to be replaced by roast potatoes, gammon, pork, cauliflower cheese, veg, more Yorkshires, stuffing and chipolatas. It's mid-week so a standard carvery costs £8.49, but if you're looking to dig an even earlier grave, you can 'eat like a King' (Henry VIII, presumably) for an extra £1.99.

It's an incongruous setting to interview one of the world's leading experts in human performance physiology, especially in the realm of endurance. He's worked closely with two of the greatest marathon runners of all time, Paula Radcliffe and Eliud Kipchoge, and was a world-class runner himself. But I'm here to talk about his pioneering work using nitrates to boost performance. It's not on the Toby menu but I'm here to discover more about the wonders of beetroot.

'Ahh, there's a car with a personalised registration number, AMJ,' I say to myself. In my head. 'That must be Andrew Jones.' It is, though I never did find out what the 'M' stood for. Maybe 'Money' by the look of Jones' car, which is an Aston Martin. 'There's clearly a few quid in Beet It,' I say tactlessly, referring to the shots that have been popular with endurance athletes for years. I knew Jones was Mr Beetroot and always thought he'd capitalised on his research through that concentrated juice. 'Nope, nothing to do with Beet It,' Jones corrects me. 'Beet It was formed by James White Drinks after we published our first studies. I have no vested interest in nitrate being effective or otherwise.' Which is great, as this insight into the power of the root will be more independent than I'd anticipated.

Apart from vitamins for health, I'm not really a supplement taker for performance. I'm a fan of caffeine, though that's in coffee form and the occasional energy gel on a ride. I tried creatine as a teenager, seeking broader shoulders and bigger biceps, but was put off by the tingling of the skin that creatine sometimes causes. More recently, I tried my son's pre-workout powder. Big mistake. We were on holiday in Whitby and I'd enjoyed an ale or two with my father the previous evening. I woke to a mild headache and an 18-year-old lad who insisted we do a weights session together at the local gym, but only after he'd mixed me his potion. Never again as it felt like my face was peeling off. I looked like I was permanently embarrassed and my cheeks itched. I think one of the ingredients was beta-alanine, which could have been partly responsible. That and the local ale nearly finished me off. I'd also played around with sodium bicarbonate, as mentioned, when showing Lawson Craddock how to time trial.

Over the years, as a long-time cycling writer, I'd seen supplements come and go, marketing teams ultimately failing to find the independent research they'd based their 40 per cent faster, longer and easier claims on. When it came to beetroot, however, my interest had remained piqued since Jones' first study back in 2009[24], which showed a 16 per cent increase in time-to-exhaustion during high-intensity exercise. Beetroot, it seemed, had transformed them into a runaway train that simply wouldn't run out of steam. I thought those figures were probably high, but beetroot never went away. The studies would keep on coming, saying that it improved endurance performance. I'd spend time with teams and there would always be a jug of deep-red smoothie for riders to consume. And recently I'd been chatting to Kevin Sprouse, director of medicine and science at EF Education–EasyPost who I'd previously asked about Whoop (more on this in Chapter 7) and asked him if the American team used it.

'Absolutely. We've used it for years, whether it's beetroot juice or concentrated beet supplements. I remember a few years ago we were at a hotel and all the riders kept on getting beets from the salad bar.

It kept being emptied and the guys were peed off as there were none left. It's not a fad that blew away; that said, even without the nitrate thing, it's still a delicious, healthy food.'

Jones and I enter the Kingdom of Calories and I start by asking him to explain the mechanics of this 'nitrate thing'.

'The first thing that's worth mentioning is that beetroot's just a vehicle,' he says. 'There's nothing magical about beetroot per se, it's the nitrate in it. You can get nitrate from rocket, spinach, radishes and all sorts of other foods, most of them from Dart's Farm [a popular Devonian farm shop] just down the road.

'When you eat or drink nitrate-containing food, it goes into your stomach and then your intestine. Some of the nitrate then crosses the intestinal wall to your blood, but also into your entero-salivary system. Over the next few hours, salivary glands secrete nitrate-rich saliva into your mouth. The bacteria in your mouth then metabolises nitrate, breaking it down into nitrite. Now you're swallowing nitrite into your stomach. This then gets into your intestine and into your blood. So, you have nitrite and nitrate concentrations in your blood, which are elevated and travelling around your body all the time.'

The nitrite is then converted to nitric oxide in the gut, causing among things your blood vessels to widen, which means exercise becomes easier, you can work harder and, voilà, you've won the Tour. Or something like that. 'That's the accepted explanation but there also seems to be an effect in the skeletal muscle cells themselves, leading to the actual energy cost of exercise being a little lower when you've ingested nitrate. Your power relative to VO_2 max is a little lower so you should be able to keep going longer at that intensity before you're exhausted.'

While many athletes might use beetroot juice on a daily basis, Jones says taking it acutely is fine, meaning quaffing a shot before a decent ride rather than all the time. 'Nitrite concentration peaks after around two to three hours. You can take it chronically but it doesn't store that well in the body.'

Concentrated shots are arguably better than the root veg because you'd need so many roots to match the nitrates in a small shot. What's more, the vegetables are high in fibre, which as we've learned, is not what pro riders want during races. Not having to take a hit of the concentrated form every day is financially good news, as they don't come especially cheap. And there's further good news to come.

'The consensus is that the recreational athlete benefits more than elite athletes. A meta-analysis of studies suggests that if your VO_2 max is greater than 65ml/min/kg, the effects are pretty small.' I'm nearer 50ml/min/kg, so I'll be ordering immediately, especially when Jones delivers the cherry on the cake.

'You're doing the Étape? Are there climbs over 2000m?' 'Too many,' I reply. 'There's evidence that nitrates benefit you more at altitude. When the air thins, your arterial oxygen saturation levels drop. What you found with nitrates is that because it lowers your metabolic rate, those oxygen saturations levels are preserved. That'll pay off for a one-off event like the Étape but not for a training camp because your body won't have the stimulus to release the EPO that produces red blood cells, so will hamper adaptation.' (More on altitude in Chapter 10.)

So, imbibing beetroot juice leads to an improvement in endurance, at altitude and, from new studies, potentially during intense sprints, too, due to the interplay between calcium and muscle generation. 'Just avoid mouthwash,' he warns. 'The anti-bacteria kills the bacteria [in your mouth and so] kills the whole process.'

I'm convinced, so I change the topic and spend the next 20 minutes asking Jones about the legend that is Kipchoge before Jones politely says he needs to leave. 'I'm meeting someone for lunch. That's why I asked to meet you here. My main role is professor at Exeter University and this place is on the way to Exmouth.'

And with that, AMJ speeds off for I suspect something more nutritious than an all-you-can-eat buffet at a Toby Carvery. In the meantime, I head straight for Amazon and order 15 x 70ml shots of Beet It Nitrate 400 (other shots are available) for £20. Thanks to Prime, they arrive the same day before I've even driven back to Bristol and I set about testing out the effects – when I can. The problem with that two- to three-hour peaking period is that most of my rides, especially on the Wattbike, are done soon after waking. However, it's fine for Sunday rides and I move a few sessions to later in the day.

The taste is surprisingly fine. And yes, it does leave your wee a deep red in no time at all. But did it make me a better cyclist? Well, if you at the back could just bring that fence over here for me to sit on, that'd be grand. In all honesty, I don't know; I don't have empirical data to say yes, I rode 8 per cent longer or I rode the same distance for 8 per cent less energy. However, and this could be the wonderful world of the placebo effect, I did sense a slight improvement. Whether this was the knock-on effect of drinking the shots that kept at the forefront of my mind the importance of good nutrition, which meant I was making better food choices, who knows. I didn't hit the labs, didn't let Iñigo San-Millán take my blood and didn't undertake power tests directly pre- and directly post-beet, but I can see what Jones meant on mentioning a social-media group he was a part of. 'I'm in a Facebook group called Three-Hour Marathon Runner', he told me. 'I'm amazed at how much positive spiel there is about beetroot juice. To be honest, the anecdotal is actually stronger than the data evidence.'

Ultimately, all I can conclude is the same as Sprouse – even if it's not the endurance golden ticket some claim, it certainly does no harm (unless of course you're sensitive to nitrites, in which case avoid it at all costs). Which is more than I can say about my son's pre-workout powder.

As for how the rest of my training's going, by mid- to late May I'm over four months into the programme, so there is less than two months to go until L'Étape du Tour on Sunday, 10 July. I remain married to the Wattbike and the weekly long ride's now up to the four-hour mark. One ride in particular hammered home how joyful the simple act of cycling can be. I loaded my bike with gels and energy bars and rode to Somerset's Chew Valley and beyond. The sun had her most glorious hat on and it was early on a Sunday, so the country roads were appreciatively quiet. Birds tweeted and the smell of wild garlic permeated the air (which, as an aside, I thought was growing rather late in the season. Many years ago, I became obsessed by the stuff. My family never again want to see, let alone taste, my wild garlic soup). It was bucolic bliss on a bike, made even more enjoyable by actually feeling fitter and, I hesitate to say it, lighter. I was no sub-60kg climber but I'd dropped to 87–87.5kg, depending on which side of the scale I stood on. (The left was on a creaky floorboard, the right side on a firm floorboard!) This was 5kg lighter than January, which might not sound much, but it was noticeable on my Vitus. As I eased on to the drops – which I could manage for increasingly longer stretches after my wind-tunnel take-home (more in Chapter 6) – I felt less of a midriff drop on to the top tube. In layman's talk, my stomach was less bulbous, meaning it was less impeding for a cleaner pedalling stroke. Yes, there remained nerves aplenty at the thought of the triple whammy of Galibier, Croix de Fer and Alpe d'Huez, but with Kier's fuelling advice and a gallon of beetroot juice to fuel my engine, I felt that little bit closer to if not taming at least completing the biggest physical challenge of my life. All I had to do was to keep on breathing easy...

9

Suffocating Stamina

T-minus one month

It's Wednesday 15 June 2022 and a heatwave has flirted with the UK, leaving lawns parched and drivers restless, especially the 400-word-a-minute Romanian lady who's Ubering (is Ubering a verb? It is now) me to Bristol Airport. There's little air in the atmosphere or within this suffocating taxi as a crash ahead has left me static, sweaty and stressed.

A day with Ineos Grenadiers in Andorra is the destination. Currently, that seems a lifetime away as many logistical hurdles await, and not just whether I'll make my flight in time. I'm meeting my chauffer/world-leading cycling coach at 9 a.m. on the Thursday to uncover why WorldTour teams are increasingly heading to higher climes in search of higher performance and to see if I can apply any oxygen-depleted, performance-boosting advice to my own training plan. My flight's at 7 p.m., to arrive at 10 p.m. Barcelona (Airport) time once you add on that hour difference. Car hire closes at 11 p.m. It all needs to run smoother than Guardiola's tiki-taka style of football circa 2011 to land, disembark, negotiate passport control Brexit style and scuttle off to my yellow-sticker car choice, aka the most affordable. Inevitably, this means the smallest vehicle for a relatively large man. Any delay and Enterprise will be closed, not to reopen until 8 a.m. It's a three-hour drive to Andorra, meaning I'd miss my 9 a.m. altitude education were that to happen. The negativity deepens on realising my accommodation's miles away from the airport. Budgets are tight – hence that toy car – so I could do without a further taxi.

These are my thoughts, which, unlike the Uber, are running away with me. Of course, the driver is blissfully unaware of my rising cortisol levels as she chats away to me.

'We are moving…' I snap back into focus, rush through departure, wait at gate 10, my anxiety climbing as the flight is delayed by 30 minutes. Thankfully, after much on-board fidgeting, and on disembarking being directed to the incorrect Catalan passport control queue, I arrive at the Barcelona Enterprise car hire with 10 minutes to spare, hot, dripping and fatigued. But the car is ready, as is the standard line of every European car hire company I've ever used when covering cycling races and training camps abroad. 'Your excess is £1500. If the merest scratch scars our fleet, we'll kidnap your family, burn your village, and spread disease and pestilence over every inch of your land.' My word. 'Thankfully' – a grin replaces the grimace – 'for just £50, you can save your country and future from rack and ruin.'

The microscopic detail with which Mr Catalan-on-Commission inspects every inch of the car convinces me that it'll be £50 well spent. To top it all, the fuel policy is return as found rather than full-to-full, meaning a volume guessing game on return, which inevitably means overfilling to stave off any further fines. 'I'm sure Egan Bernal and co don't have to go through this,' I ponder as I arrive at my hostel. (In my rush to book, I'd inadvertently added an extra 's' to the word 'hotel' and wondered why it was the most affordable stay near the airport. Thankfully, there are no teenage backpackers in my dorm. Still, knowing I have to be up at 5 a.m., I sleep poorly, but it matters not: I'm away on time.)

The early morning sun is still strong enough to leave a heat haze on the N-1411 to Andorra. There's also a hazy silhouette of mountains up ahead, which I suspect is Andorra. Or a Bob Ross painting. Either way, I'm cruising along, alone aside from the pine trees that perfume both sides and the steps of vegetation that ascend ahead of the jagged rock face. Time passes, my mind wanders and before I know it, I'm parked up outside the Golden Tulip hotel in Andorra la Vella, and being picked up by Ineos Grenadiers' coach Adrian Lopez, who directly trains Laurens de Plus, Cameron Wurf, Andrey Amador and Jhonatan Narváez.

'Welcome,' Spaniard Lopez greets me. 'We just need to nip into my apartment in La Massana to pick up some wheels.' La Massana's a short drive from Andorra la Vella, from where we'll follow Ben Tulett. The team has an altitude camp the following month, which I was invited to. However, I'll be too busy facing my own mountains (the Étape), so I opt for solo assessment.

Ben Tulett, a 20-year-old from Sevenoaks, England, is new to the team this season. Like the protagonists we came across in Chapter 3 – the likes of teammate Tom Pidcock, Wout van Aert and Mathieu van der Poel – Tulett's move came off the back of a strong reputation forged off-road. He won the Junior World Cyclo-cross Championships two years in a row (2018 and 2019), plus the National U23 Championships in 2020. His road CV's not too shabby, either, Tulett winning the National Junior Championships in 2018. In the senior ranks, he finished fifth overall at the Tour of Antalya 2020.

'We'll meet Ben en route,' Lopez says after dropping a pair of wheels along with musettes on the back seat of the team's Mercedes-Benz E220. 'Often that'll happen as, unlike Monaco, where many of the team are based, Andorra's much bigger. Jonathan [Castroviejo] and Tao [Geoghegan Hart] are 30 minutes away in different directions. Anyway, it shouldn't take too long to catch Ben as the main focus of today's ride is cresting Port d'Envalira. It's 27.5km long and reaches an altitude of around 2500m. The average gradient's not too bad, though, at around 5%.'

'27.5km long?!' I retort with a statement that demands both question mark and exclamation mark. 'Are there any other climbs comparable to this in Europe?'

'Few,' Adrian replies. 'I guess the one that jumps out is the Galibier. It's in this year's Tour de France.'

And this year's L'Étape du Tour. Rollocks!

'Ahh, there's Ben now.' Adrian points. Ben's in the orange livery of Ineos' training kit rather than the red and blue of racing. It's rather sharp, both visually and commercially, the British team's marketing department taking a cue from football and merchandising as many kits as loyalty affords.

Ben's sub-60kg frame and cheeks that look shaved of bum fluff rather than stubble makes me feel old. He looks younger than my 18-year-old son.

'Just stick to tempo,' Adrian advises Ben. 'It's a hard climb and this isn't a hard day.'

With that and a degree of spittle draped over his right cheek, Ben continues while we drive behind. Adrian spends a lot of time shadowing the glutes of the world's best cyclists alone, the silence occasionally broken by offering snippets of training advice through the passenger window. It affords us the time to take a dive into why Andorra's become the epicentre of altitude training.

'It's been shown that you need to head over 1500m to "enjoy" the benefits of altitude training, though the closer you get to around 2000–2200m, the better. Too low and the stress will be insufficient for the body to stimulate the increased EPO that the riders are after; too high and training intensity will be too low. That's why riders come to Andorra.'

Cycling stalwarts will be all too aware of EPO or erythropoietin. This hormone is naturally made by your kidneys to trigger your bone marrow to make red blood cells. The idea of 'training high' is that by exposing yourself to an environment low in oxygen (more specifically, a lower partial pressure, or the pressure of a gas in a mixture comprising two or more gases, of oxygen – oxygen percentage is constant but the fall in atmospheric pressure decreases the partial pressure of oxygen, effectively meaning that you get less when you breathe in), the body will adapt by increasing red blood cell count and so become a furnace for burning oxygen to power the working muscles. And as WorldTour road cycling is predominantly an endurance event, where oxygen rules, the result is an improvement in performance, both in the mountains and back down at sea level. Of course, EPO is created in the lab, too, as we discovered in Chapter 4. That's a no-no. Altitude training's a yes, though interestingly not the use of altitude tents in Italy under a law related to public health and artificially boosting performance (more on that later).

There's another physiological reason altitude is seen as a road-cycling panacea – studies show that training at altitude increases aerobic capacity (VO$_2$ max) by 3–8 per cent; lowers heart rate, both at rest and during exercise; elevates levels of myoglobin, the muscle protein; and reduces lactic acid build-up, so you can pedal harder for longer.

On paper, altitude training's a no-brainer. In reality… 'It doesn't work for all as some riders are responders and feel good, while some are non-responders, feel bad and just don't adapt in the same way,' Adrian explains.

Before heading to Andorra, I'd read a study in the journal *Medicine & Science in Sports & Exercise*[25] highlighting the benefits of being born in Bogotá (elevation 2640m) rather than Bognor Regis (elevation 5m). The team, led by David Barranco-Gil of the European University of Madrid, analysed power data of three pro teams between 2013 and 2020 to see if there were differences between those born at altitudes above 1798m compared to those born and raised closer to sea level, especially during mountain stages.

There were many. One of the key differentiators between altitude natives and lowlanders was the former group's greater capacity to maintain higher levels of oxygen in their blood during exercise in the mountains; in other words, they were more efficient at grabbing whatever oxygen is available in the lungs to diffuse into the blood. Despite the 'low' group training often at altitude, they just couldn't match the genetic and environmental development of the 'high' group.

'How does Ben cope?' I ask Adrian.

'He's relatively new to altitude training so we're still working that one out.' He agrees with the Barranco-Gil research to a degree, though he suggests the likes of Tulett have greater bandwidth to grow.

'It's tricky as the South Americans, like [Egan] Bernal and [Richard] Carapaz, are natives of altitudes of more than 2000m, so when they altitude train in Europe, the aim's about keeping their adaptations rather than improving them. The fact Ben's so young, if he can cope with the added atmospheric pressures, he'll do well.'

This 'coping' (or not) is fed back via anecdotal reports. However, given the modern empirical world of road cycling, I ask whether Ineos has delved deeper than just a conversation. 'Of course,' Adrian replies. 'Every day we use a pulse oximeter to measure the saturation of oxygen in the blood. If you're 98 per cent at sea level, that might drop to 92 per cent when you start training at altitude. How the rider feels with that drop is very much an individual response – they might feel fine, they might feel terrible. But as time at altitude progresses, that figure should rise as they adapt.

'The riders also have blood tests at the start and end of camp with most adaptations having happened within 20 days. But this isn't all about oxygen intake. One of the most important changes is how a rider copes psychologically with the lower atmospheric pressure at high altitude and the perceived threat. The Grand Tours always hit mountains above 2000m and if your brain's not used to it, you can haemorrhage time. In the last 6km of a big climb, if you're [down by] two seconds per kilometre and then 12 seconds in the last kilometre, plus time lost to your competitor because of bonuses, that's over 30 seconds [you've lost]. That could make or break your race.'

Ben continues to knock out a metronomic cadence and pace and a power output of around 260 watts, while I play spot the professional. According to Adrian, over 70 WorldTour riders now use Andorra as their European base and I've just seen two of them fly past: George Bennett of UAE Team Emirates and Luke Durbridge of Team BikeExchange. Then a streak of pink flashes by. 'That's Magnus Cort [of EF Education–EasyPost],' Adrian says. 'Many riders will be here all year round, though they'll hit the likes of Mallorca and Calpe for December and January training camps. Many of the mountain-top finishes are closed to cyclists then because of snow.'

This perma-living high is proving popular and is down to what Primož Roglič's coach, Mathieu Heijboer, calls the 'accumulation of altitude'. I acted as compere to Heijboer's presentation one year at the annual Science & Cycling Conference in exchange for free entry. The former pro, who's now performance director at Jumbo–Visma, coined the term after Roglič and Heijboer had spent seven weeks at altitude in Tignes, France, just before the 2021 Tour de France. Roglič and his team had already endured breathless sessions in Tenerife and Sierra Nevada earlier in the season. Unfortunately, Roglič didn't get the chance to ascertain whether those weeks spent up high would result in the top step in Paris as he crashed and withdrew.

'There's evidence that repeated altitude camps, during a single season or across multiple seasons, means that the body is exposed to hypoxia a number of times a year, which is more beneficial in terms of increasing red blood cell count than just a single camp in a year,' Heijboer explained. 'It's like doing one long ride at the weekend versus lots of slightly shorter rides in the week.'

Not only that, but riders can often train to a higher quality at later camps. This is down to what scientists call a 'hypoxic memory', which enables them to acclimatise more quickly to altitude at subsequent camps, allowing a higher quality of training (with greater volume and/ or intensity), which means the overall training stimulus is heightened.

But there is a balance to be had. 'We'll often drive or ride to the Spanish side for low-altitude work,' Adrian says. 'From a mechanical point of view, you can work harder.' And that's important, he adds, because while high altitude can result in blood parameter improvements that are conducive to a more proficient cardiovascular system, a low-oxygen environment can actually weaken muscles. This, it transpires, is due to the hypoxic melting pot triggering a rider's adrenal glands to increase cortisol production. Cortisol is a catabolic hormone, meaning it breaks down muscle for energy. High cortisol levels cause the rider's body to morph from a muscle-building state to one of muscle breakdown.

It's his job to pinpoint the physiological sweet spot between oxygen-rich blood and powerful muscles via software like TrainingPeaks and old-school talking to the rider. It's part science, part art, but experience tells Lopez that young prospects like Tulett need to be handled with care.

'He is young and did fantastically well at the Giro d'Italia [finishing 38th in his first Grand Tour]. But he won't race the Vuelta a España as two three-week races in one season is too much. We need to tread step by step and see how he reacts. That said, physically I have no doubt he could handle it. But the problem is up here [Adrian points to his cropped dark hair]. We need to build mental tolerance, to help them handle an increasing amount of stress. Often, we notice the physiological stats for a rider might be similar throughout the season but their performance fades. They need rest, for the mind more than anything else.'

But not now. Tulett's still climbing, I'm still admiring the stunning mountainous scenery while at the same time sinking further back into my passenger seat with the thought of tackling similar in France. As the drive continues and conversation begins to dry up, I'm increasingly filling moments of silence by repeating, 'It's beautiful here', in a faux Spanish accent that harks of Steve McClaren's tenure at Twente when he applied a Dutch brogue to slowed-down pidgin English. Adrian politely ignores my geological gushing and instead delivers a history lesson.

'There's a dark past to this place. It remained neutral in World War II and acted as a smuggling route from Spain into France. But there are tales of Andorran people becoming rich by killing people for their gold as they passed through. This is the real history of Andorra.'

Blimey. I didn't expect that. Does that explain why Andorra's one of the richest places in Europe? My research couldn't corroborate Adrian's tales of the killing fields. And on the positive, they're incredibly receptive to cyclists, waiting and letting them pass when time and space allows. It's a nation of hikers, cyclists, skiers and runners.

'Andorra is an independent principality but I'd say it's more French than Spanish.' Adrian has softened his tour of Andorra slightly to talk politics. 'The prime minister [Xavier Zamora] is Andorran but arguably he holds less power than the "co-princes of Andorra". These two heads of state are [Emmanuel] Macron, the French president, and the other is a Roman Catholic guy who's high up in the Vatican.'

This 'Roman Catholic guy' is Archbishop Joan-Enric Vives, who's the current Bishop of Urgell. Back in 1278, this landlocked microstate was founded by a treaty between the then bishop and the County of Foix (in what is now southern France). Ever since, the Bishop of Urgell has retained their place at the head of the Andorran table.

All I knew before that nervy flight from Bristol was that England beat Andorra in two qualifiers for the 2022 World Cup and, thanks to a swift search on Encyclopaedia Britannica, this is a cyclist's heartland thanks to a cluster of mountain valleys whose streams unite to form the Gran Valira River. Two of these streams, the Madriu and the Perafita, flow into the Madriu-Perafita-Claror Valley, which occupies about 1/10th of Andorra's land area and is characterised by glacial landscapes, steep valleys and open pastures. The valley was designated a UNESCO World Heritage Site in 2004.

'We've reached the summit!' exclaims Adrian, returning things to the present. And what an ugly present it turns out to be. We pull over in a huge gravel car park, next to which sit not one but two petrol stations – Shell and Elf. It's an underwhelming destination at the highest road pass in the Pyrenees region, so I do a 180 to remind myself of the beauty that's just passed, just as Ben arrives (we'd overtaken him a couple kilometres earlier).

'How are you feeling now,' I ask? The spittle from earlier is now nestled on Ben's upper lip.

'Not bad but as it gets higher, it becomes much harder. Living in the UK, you clearly don't have access to these climbs though I guess it's still just turning pedals. But it's a cycling paradise and an amazing place to live and train.'

Ben chows down on an energy bar and looks more drained than he did earlier. 'My body still has to adapt,' he continues. 'I'm sure it will the longer I'm here.'

One thing I've learned on my journey so far is that long solo rides can become boring. (With around a month to go until L'Étape, on one of those long weekly rides I reflect that joining a cycling club might have been prudent. Next time…) Yes, they're great for burning fat, strengthening lungs and heart, and becoming at one with a saddle, but that's hard to keep at the forefront of your mind when you're stuck with yourself for hours on end.

I'm not in a minority as I notice a wireless earphone in Ben's left ear. 'It's just a little bit of background music to keep me active. Anything with a good beat works, especially drum and bass. It's always nicer to ride with teammates, which will become a greater option as the team wants to build an Andorran base. Training with others pushes you harder and is more motivating. That said, sometimes it's just nice to head out the door.'

Or home. After a brief conflab with Adrian, they decide to curtail today's ride as Ben's not feeling great. The Giro's not that long gone plus the altitude is starting to chafe. He's heading back to the UK the following week to race the national championships, so there's no need to push on when the mind and body are telling him to pull back. Just as Ben prepares to descend whence we just came, I notice a black band on his left wrist.

'What's that?'

'It's a wristband with the hashtag "Ride for Charlie" written on,' Ben replies, tentatively. 'It's for Charlie Craig.' This is a small, often tragic, world. This is the Charlie Craig who died in his sleep at the age of 15 and whose father, Nick, I interviewed at the National Cyclo-cross Championships earlier in the year (*see* Chapter 3). 'Me and Charlie were best friends and used to race against each other all the time. I'm still close to Charlie's family and am wearing this to raise funds for a cardiac machine to scan children. For me, Charlie remains a huge motivation to work as hard as I can. It's five years since he passed...' Ben tails off. It's all just all incredibly sad.

Adrian and I drive back down the hill to where the ride started. It's been an informative, entertaining, emotional and, of course, beautiful morning. And one that I would look to replicate the next day by renting a bike. I question these good intentions later that day as I drive the same climb in my overpriced, undersized rental car. The heat now is stifling and, after exiting my car and walking small sections near the top, I'm left breathless, due to both the rarefied air and that hypnotic panorama. Slowly but surely over the past five months, the consistent training, the hint of weight loss, the learnings from the professionals and my own one-on-one advice had built belief, and had made me feel that completing L'Étape du Tour 2022 would soon radiate on my palmarès. Remember the life-affirming wild-garlic glow of Chapter 8? On this sweltering afternoon in Andorra, that glow was snuffed out. My house of confident cards had collapsed. How the hell am I going to conquer the Étape, which starts with a mountain of this grandeur followed by two more?

'Adrian, are there any other routes you can recommend?' I WhatsApp. 'Here's a PDF of the area,' he swiftly messages back. The map features 21 routes – more specifically, climbs – that all look upsetting. There's Sant Julià de Lòria to Coll de la Gallina, 12.2km, rising 1019m at an average gradient of 8.4%. Or I can choose a different form of execution from Sant Julià de Lòria and climb 17.4km, rising 1127m at a gradient of 6.5%. Or why not go for the 10.5km, 6.9% ascent from El Serrat to Arcalís? Hmm, bullet, guillotine or noose?

I drive back to the Golden Tulip hotel and ponder the next day's possible ride while grabbing a bite to eat. The centre of Andorra la Vella is a world away from the white flowers, purple hues, pine-fresh ambience of earlier in the day. It resembles one large duty free with tackiness around every turn. Around another turn are Dan Martin and his wife, Jess, who maintain this as their base despite Dan retiring in 2021. Dan still packs a punch and walks out of sight before I can ask him for culinary recommendations. The last time I interviewed Dan, he revealed how he part-owned a restaurant chain in London called Frog, run by Adam Handling, who reached the final of *MasterChef: The Professionals* in 2013. But he's gone, so I choose a chicken kebab with one sauce.

And that was mission Andorra complete. 'What about the following day's bike ride?' you ask. Well, for such a bike-loving country – I even saw them setting up for a round of the UCI Mountain Bike World Cup the following month – road bikes were thin on the ground. 'Why didn't you sort this when you were back in the UK?' you could well enquire. And you'd be right to ask. This was an opportune moment to really ride on the shoulders of giants. But again, I point that finger of blame at life tampering with my (often lack of) organisational skills.

I'd been so delighted to spend time with the Ineos Grenadiers, a team with whom it's hard work to organise one-on-one time beyond media days, I'd failed to pencil in an altitude ride to challenge my own performance. In all honesty, I'd also thought it would be easy to just turn up and hire a bike. As it transpired, I was wrong. I called in to one bike shop, which only rented out mountain bikes. After looking me up and down, the employee recommended an e-mountain bike. 'I'll leave it, thank you.' I then found a bike shop that did rent out road bikes. 'Presumably, you want an e-bike,' the chap asked? Cheeky beggars. This didn't fill me with confidence. What had they seen? 'No, a standard road will be absolutely fine,' I replied, hammering home the 'absolutely' as if my life depended on it. 'Oh, we don't have any available. So, it's e-bike or nothing?' 'How much?' 'Around €250 for the day.' I looked at my bank account. Nothing it is.

I can't feel my penis.

Bristol is 11m above sea level. That's little higher than a molehill, so I'd chosen to head east to London's Altitude Centre to sample the delights of Andorran air within a stone's throw of St Paul's Cathedral. I'd experienced simulated altitude once before many years ago when an altitude tent company had sent me one on loan. You place it over your bed – it took an age to set up and the generator that sucked air out of the bedroom sounded like, well, a generator sucking air out of the bedroom. Needless to say, after my wife and I had endured a couple of loud, sleepless nights, the tent went, and I nobly sacrificed bucketloads of EPO for my marriage.

Now, I'm 30 minutes into a Wattbike session, dialled into the oxygen level you'd experience at a nose-bleeding 2700m and the altitude's apparently meddling with my appendage. I don't know whether it's lack of oxygen reaching so far down or the saddle, but any thoughts of adding more children to our existing two (I don't have any – I'm not insane) are disappearing with every pedal stroke. Thankfully, once the session ends, the blood flow restarts and all is as nature intended.

'The first thing to say is that nothing can match an altitude camp,' explains the centre's manager Sam Rees. 'But few people can afford the time and money to spend weeks on end at altitude. This is the next best thing.'

It's also easier to quantify the results, as though altitude camps are seen as the pinnacle, it's difficult to unpick exactly how much improvement derives from oxygen-deprived adaptations and how much is simply down to having a focused block of training with support staff on hand to deal with your every whim.

The Altitude Centre was founded in 2003 and in the intervening years has forged an impressive client list, including former world heavyweight boxing champion Anthony Joshua, double Olympic triathlon gold medallist Alistair Brownlee, England's national rugby union team and numerous Premier League clubs, including Liverpool, Aston Villa and Tottenham Hotspur. Arguably, its bread and butter, though, is mountaineers.

'Whoever uses our facilities has the option of booking sessions here or buying or renting a machine off us,' says Rees. 'As long as they're consistent with it, they can be pretty much assured of at least a 2 per cent boost in performance.'

I won't be consistent with it as I don't live in London. But many are, heading over to Trump Street for a lunchtime workout *sans* oxygen. Or they were until Covid struck. With office workers their core audience, their business has been slow to return to pre-pandemic levels. But they're getting there, says Rees. I've numerous maximal gains to seek before truly justifying regular altitude sessions, but I thought I'd enjoy – endure – a sampler. If I were to book a block, it would be worth it as it becomes clear I'd probably cope better than the likes of Pogačar and co. 'Reports state that the fitter you are, you almost cope less well at altitude because your body is hugely efficient and extracts all the oxygen,' says Rees. 'That can leave some individuals light of head.'

Higher, Unfitter, Stronger, that's my motto.

Rees sets me up in the altitude chamber, which is a square room about 5m x 5m. There are a further three Wattbikes, four treadmills, a

Concept2 rower and two powerbags (20kg and 10kg). Three TV screens are attached in front, one of which displays my data – average power, heart rate, duration, oxygen saturation – while two others market the Altitude Centre. There's a fridge full of mineral water, plus a generator. It's a cool industrial aesthetic with steel beams above, a cable network of lights and floor-to-ceiling mirrors, ensuring I can view my deterioration from every direction. There's also dance music.

All that's left to do is pedal. Which I do. And for 30 minutes I don't know what the fuss is about. I'm hot but my heart rate's a manageable 150bpm and all is fine, apart from a hint of sickness stemming from eating a cheese-and-onion pasty on the train up. (Note to self: manage eating on the fly much better than currently. Learn from Flanders!)

Then things change, and quite dramatically. Around 36 minutes in, I can feel the energy drain from my body. Five minutes later, I'm practising a deep-breathing technique taught to me by a Scandinavian physiotherapist at the now-disbanded Tinkoff team on a writing gig, which essentially involves consciously taking deeper breaths through your mouth and aggressive exhaling through the nose. Apparently, it engages the diaphragm more. But it doesn't help. The descent into fatigue due to the ascent into altitude is stark and I'm glad it's just a 45-minute session. As I shower, my legs wobble with that jelly-legged feeling synonymous with triathlon in the bike-to-run transition. And then, of course, there was the penis problem.

I soon recover but the experience has been another anxious altitude shot in the arm for what lies ahead at the Étape. Questions churn around my brain. 'How will this 45-year-old mind and body cope with three mountains of around 2000m?' 'Is there anything I can do to affordably simulate the Galibier from Bristol?' 'What if my penis drops off?'

'Just make sure your iron levels are topped up before you go,' says Rees. 'It's a real struggle at altitude if they're not.'

Back in Bristol, I'm fruitlessly searching for ways to mimic the mountains at home and come across ITV's *Chris Boardman: The Final Hour* on YouTube[26]. It documents Boardman's journey en route to breaking Eddy Merckx's 28-year-old hour record by just 10m. That was back in 2000. The documentary offers an insight into marginal gains to come.

It includes a clip where the camera pans to Boardman's Wirral home. 'What we have here is my son George's bedroom that I've converted into a hypoxic chamber,' he describes in his distinctive, warm Liverpudlian tones. 'All the windows are completely sealed with tape. The door is completely sealed with tape. There are three tubes coming in, which are linked to generators in the workshop outside and they pump in oxygen at 16 per cent compared to the normal 21 per cent. We're at the equivalent of 15,000 feet now.' Boardman's then filmed pedalling away on his ergometer, sweating profusely over poor George's carpet.

It's fascinating. And completely impractical.

Instead, I purchase an altitude mask – the cheapest I can for £25 – based off potentially spurious claims of stimulating the effects of high-altitude training. I use the muzzle for a couple of Wattbike sessions and just find it incredibly uncomfortable, akin to a fitness test. But with the fitness tests I've endured, at least I could see a path to progression. This just appears to inhibit my breathing rate.

'In answer to your question, no, there's no evidence that they mimic altitude at all.' That's James Barber of the Altitude Centre. Barber is their lead performance specialist and has a masters with first-class honours in physiology. I'd emailed him for his thoughts. 'The key to altitude is that it alters the partial pressure of oxygen, which is the product of the overall air pressure (barometric pressure) and the oxygen concentration within that air. At terrestrial altitude, barometric pressure is reduced, whereas hypoxic generators that simulate altitude reduce the oxygen concentration in normobaric air [normal barometric pressure, as found at sea level]. So-called "elevation masks" do neither and so do not simulate altitude – so much so that they have often been rebranded as "training masks". I'd argue they actually reduce the quality of workout.'

Many wouldn't. But the mask is not for me. I pop the mask away in my sports drawer, never to be seen again. I research a little more and think about tackling my next problem.

The effort at the Altitude Centre left me saturated, raspberry red and puffing out of every orifice; in fact, when I play back my recording for transcription purposes, there's such unsettling wheezing that I feel like handing myself in to the police. But I refrain as not long after, on a late June Monday, I'm at the Porsche Human Performance Lab in Silverstone in search of heat rather than altitude. The reasons are twofold. The first is obvious: L'Étape du Tour takes place in mid-July in the south-west of France where roadside temperatures could easily surpass 40°C. The second is altitude related and links to a 2016 study I came across in the journal *Frontiers of Physiology* (I know how to have a good time!) entitled 'Cross Acclimation between Heat and Hypoxia'[27], which was undertaken by academics at Coventry University, UK. With little time to spare, I went straight to the conclusion, which read: 'Heat acclimation improved cellular and systemic physiological tolerance to steady-state exercise in moderate hypoxia. Additionally, we show for the first time that heat acclimation improved cycling time trial performance to a magnitude similar to that achieved by hypoxic acclimation.'

In essence, it's saying that training in the heat not only prepares you for racing in the heat *but at altitude too*. Interest piqued, I invested the time the article deserved and read the whole thing. Twenty-one volunteers were split into three groups: heat training at 40°C; altitude training at 14 per cent oxygen, which corresponded to around 3300m; and a control group. Each group undertook 10 days of 60-minute cycling sessions at a moderate pace corresponding to 50 per cent of VO_2 max, with a series of tests including a 16km cycling time trial at an effective elevation of 3048m before and after the training period.

The results? The control group averaged 30 seconds slower on their second test, while the heat group and altitude group bettered their original efforts by 2.02 minutes and 3.16 minutes, respectively. As expected, the hypoxia group enjoyed the greatest improvements because they were training specifically for the conditions. But the hotties enjoyed a significant boost, too.

After analysing the subjects' blood, they suggested that this joint improvement was down to the rather dramatic 'heat shock proteins'.

Despite their name, they're produced under any stress. The more frequently your body's placed under stress, the greater your resting levels, which ultimately better prepares your body for heat and altitude than simply training at normal temperatures and sea level.

I've shown that altitude training at home's a tricky one. But heat? Our extortionate energy bills show that the family love pushing the thermostat to its limits.

It's why I'm now at the home of British motorsport. While wealthy middle-aged businessmen with paunches and rosé cheeks take their newly bought Porsches for a spin around the track – a reward for purchasing – this less-wealthy middle-aged writer with a decreasing paunch and soon-to-be burning cheeks is chatting to one of the lab's sport and exercise scientists, Jack Wilson. I'd played the media card once more and would endure a gratis heat session. Wilson smiles as he explains what lies ahead.

'You'll be on the Wattbike for 30 minutes, cycling at a power output we know you're comfortable at with the dial cranked up to around 40°C,' Wilson explains. Thirty minutes? That sounds optimistic. I'd ridden in a heat chamber once before in the build-up to the 2008 Beijing Olympics when I was editing a triathlon magazine, so that I could experience what endurance athletes would face in China. The test was curtailed early as my core temperature, measured by an e-pill I'd swallowed earlier, went through the roof. My torturer during that experiment, Dr Simon Hodder of Loughborough University, had soon aborted my ride, wheeled out an industrial-sized fan and planted me in front of it.

'It was a slightly lower temperature [than the one I'm about to endure] but the humidity was 80 or 90 per cent if I remember rightly,' I tell Jack, shuddering at the memory. 'I felt like I couldn't breathe.'

'Don't worry, the humidity's much lower in there,' he says. 'It's more akin to European hot days than Asian ones. And take some comfort as it could go up to 50°C, which is what many Formula One drivers have to cope with.'

About 60 per cent of their client base is from the world of motorsport with the remaining 40 per cent a mix of cyclists, runners and triathletes, both professional and amateur.

'Right, I'll hand you over to Emma [Payne, fellow sports scientist] now.' Emma cuts the small talk, closes the chamber door and I'm away. She pokes her head back in to remind me that she'll pop in frequently to measure my temperature. I haven't ingested an e-pill this time. Oh God, not rectal. That could be awkward and rather unpleasant for all involved, especially while pedalling on a saddle. 'I'll use a tympanic thermometer to take a measurement from inside your ear,' Emma clarifies. A dignified solution for all.

With that, I pedal. I heat up. I sweat. Emma occasionally checks I'm not on fire. And the pattern intensifies for 30 minutes. Emma regularly gauges how I feel by asking me to rate my perceived exertion out of 10. It rises, but this is gradual rather than steep. Still, the build-up of hot air from the generator and me is creating a rather suffocating experience that's akin to driving with my wife, whose internal thermostat is seemingly set lower than mine, resulting in the battle of the climate-control dials. My wife's will be on 25°C while mine nestles at 16°C. Unfortunately, I don't think car manufacturers took into account the laws of Brownian motion, ensuring I remain too hot and my wife too cold, which is a far from harmonious situation on a long drive. On the plus side here, though I'm hot, I'm not bothered, and this session's proving a double confidence booster. The training might actually be working and, though heat's a stress that'll impair performance, for me it looks like humidity is a greater issue than heat.

I shower, dress and continue to sweat, patches of perspiration speckling my back and armpits, then head upstairs for lunch. And what a lunch it is, presented in a large rectangular bento box that I slide the lid off to reveal compartments of nutritious and delicious grub: top left, seasoned chicken with a hint of skin left on; top right, asparagus with a beetroot dip; bottom left, smoked salmon with pipettes of cream cheese and dill; bottom right, slices of venison with batons of cucumber, cauliflower and carrot; and in the centre, a couple of slices of bread. Apart from the frozen butter that steadfastly refuses to spread, it's a triumph and means my energy levels begin to return as Wilson takes me through the results.

'You reached 39°C. If you'd reached 39.5°C, we'd have pulled you out as that's our limit in the heat chamber. That's when heat stress can kick in, albeit everyone's different. Some will experience warning signs at lower temperatures, some higher. And those warnings can be different. Mine is blurred vision; others describe symptoms of light-headedness and nausea, or pins and needles. If warning signs aren't heeded, it can lead to heat-exertion illness.

'Despite the constant workload, we could see it was harder in the heat,' adds Wilson. 'In the cool, we'd expect your heart rate to increase at that power output but plateau because you're comfortable at that pace. But here in the heat, it continued to rise. You reached around 167bpm, which would have been around 30bpm less in cooler climes. It's why exercise in the heat is such a big challenge, but the more you're exposed to it, the more your body will adapt. And the good thing is those adaptations happen pretty fast.'

And there are plenty of these beneficial adaptations. Just then, Abby Coleman walks in. Abby's a sports scientist and works for Precision Fuel & Hydration. She's going to provide further insight into my hot body by having me perform a sweat test. 'Abby loves talking about adaptation,' says Wilson. 'Over to you…'

'Oh, go on then,' she says. 'Well, the key adaptation is an increase in blood plasma volume, which elicits a lower heart rate, which reduces the strain on the cardiovascular system, so your perception of effort is down. In many ways that's linked to dehydration. When you dehydrate, water's pulled out of the bloodstream through sweating. Blood plasma volume decreases so less blood's pumping around the body, leading to less oxygen reaching the muscles. With repeated heat exposure, the body compensates by boosting this plasma, which helps you maintain a higher intensity than at the start of your heat training.

'Over five to 10 sessions (here in the chamber or at home) we'll also see a lowering of core body temperature and the onset of sweating is earlier. Of course, that makes hydration even more important but we'll come back to that with the sweat test.'

That's good news because, in theory, with several weeks to go until I head to France, I'll still have time to heat acclimate. I mention to

Abby my idea about cranking up the heating at home while I Wattbike away, specifically the underfloor heating in the kitchen. 'As long as you do it safely,' she warns. 'We've had all kinds of crazy ideas like cyclists running their bath with the doors closed and riding beside it on their turbo trainer. That said, one option is to ride in the kitchen and then have a bath. That's another popular one. Just ensure the bath is around 40°C as it needs to be above core temperature to stimulate the changes.'

It sounds uncomfortable but could be worth it. Research by Neil Walsh of Bangor University[28] showed that moderate exercise immediately followed by a 15-minute bath in 40°C water over six days during which bathing time rose by five minutes each day resulted in a 4 per cent improvement in 5km time trial time in the heat. As well as its acclimation benefits, Walsh also suggested a hot bath can improve glucose regulation and boost immunity. So, it seems that there are also acclimation benefits from merely having a bath, so maybe I'll just do that...

'In all honesty, the indoor training should serve you well,' Coleman adds. 'You obviously don't get much of a windchill apart from when using a fan so, in a way, it's a form of heat training.'

Music to my ears, especially as although bike-fitter (Phil) Burt recommended angling a fan at my groin to prevent chafing (see Chapter 2), I'd spent most of my sessions without said fan. 'Right, let's go and test your sweat...'

Thankfully, this is a sedentary task. After the brief bento-led revival, I'm feeling the effects of that chamber again. 'Don't worry, all you need to do is sit there with your arm out.' Coleman then places two electrodes on my arm that contain gel discs saturated with a chemical called pilocarpine before strapping them down. She then switches on the machine they're connected to, the 'sweat inducer', and an electric current flows through the wires. There's no tingle.

This charged pilocarpine stimulates localised sweat production by chemically triggering the sweat glands to produce sweat – a process that takes about five minutes. Coleman then replaces the gel discs with a sweat collector. It contains a blue dye so she can see when there's enough to be analysed. 'These are the machines used by Team DSM [on the WorldTour]. We've worked with them for a few years.'

After around 20 minutes, the dye has done its stuff. Coleman connects the collector to the analyser and after some swift calculations, it transpires I'm a moderate sodium sweater, coming in at 798mg/l, meaning I lose 798mg of sodium per litre of sweat. Very low is 200–300mg/l; very high is just over 2000mg/l. The average is about 970mg/l.

This is important because sodium plays a major role in channelling water from your bloodstream into your working muscles. It's vital for muscle contraction, too. When we sweat, we lose sodium, ergo when we sweat a lot, we lose a lot of sodium. Fail to replenish it, the theory goes, and you'll dehydrate and fade into obscurity.

But as you can see from that spectrum of figures, we're all different. Why this is so is rather interesting. 'When you start sweating and fluid passes from your blood through to the surface of your skin, it passes through the sweat glands,' Coleman explains. 'Your genetic make-up dictates how much sodium's retained. This machine was actually designed for individuals with cystic fibrosis who absorb too much sodium.'

While your sodium levels are broadly set by DNA, they can dial up or down slightly depending on diet, training status and heat acclimation. 'This is only half the equation,' Coleman continues. 'You then multiply this figure by sweat rate. From your efforts in the heat chamber, we calculated that when riding temperatures of around 40°C you'll sweat between 1.25 and 1.5 litres an hour.'

So, if I'm losing around 800mg of sodium per litre of sweat, that's around 1200mg every hour. That's where Precision's commercial arm comes in as they then prescribe sodium tablets based broadly on that figure. They have 500mg, 1000mg and 1500mg options with each fizzy pill popped in 500ml of water.

Coleman suggests the 1000mg option for the Étape and highlights that there's no way I'd manage to drink 1.5 litres an hour, every hour, on a bike, up mountains, but to at least aim for around 750ml to 1 litre. Your stomach can only cope with so much, too, before it becomes bloated and uncomfortable.

'One final thing,' she says before I head off. 'Consider sodium pre-loading with a strong electrolyte drink before the start. It'll give you a bigger reservoir to drain from when competing; a bigger buffer if you start from a high baseline before hitting the red zone.'

Back in Bristol, I order the 1500mg option too. I hope this goes down as smoothly as the Beet It shots, which I continue to quaff a few hours before most rides. Mind you, I won't be popping a 1500 tab every day, just before long rides, so I should be fine. I also purchase a bath thermometer for £3.99 and spend the next couple of weeks either indoor cycling and bathing or simply bathing, at a minimum 40°C. I crank up the underfloor heating a couple of times, as well, but with many bills to pay, I decide that's a step too far. Does it work? I'm certainly sweating more. But I'll only really know come Sunday 10 July 2022, which is inching ever closer.

Despite the lack of altitude training, I am hitting more mountains – OK, hills – on my weekly long ride. One of my regulars involves riding on the Bristol to Bath cycle path before veering off into the Roman city – and then out – via Lansdown Hill. The hill's little more than 3km long but averages a gradient of 6.8% and peaks at 12.2%. When I started this painful journey, my lungs felt like they were going to pop. Now, in June, many months down the line, there is still an anticipation of organ explosion but less physical pain. I'm still feeling a little mental anguish, however, from my Andorran eye-opener but, on a more positive note, nutritionist Emily Kier's advice alongside consistent training are having an impact on my weight, which is helping on the ascents. On the negative side, Lansdown Hill is a shallower average gradient than Alpe d'Huez and more than 13km shorter. And it hasn't come off the back off riding two further Alpine mountains. If you ask me now how I feel about my Étape du Tour chances, I'd say confused. Which many would say has been my state of being for 45 years.

Preparing to Peak (or Pass Out)

T-minus three weeks to one day

The heartbeat of the modern peloton is Sheffield. More precisely, Bonsall, Matlock, around 13km from the centre of England's fourth largest city and on the fringes of the Peak District. It sounds fanciful, doesn't it? Both Sheffield and Bonsall were forged on their industrial past – steel and mining lead, respectively. Their days at the epicentre of innovation seem behind them. There's professional cycling heritage here, too. But while county rivals Leeds and its close locales have spawned modern legends Tom Pidcock and Elizabeth Deignan, plus icons of the past, Barry Hoban and Beryl Burton, Sheffield's major claim to professional road-riding fame focuses on Malcolm Elliott, who won the points classification at the 1989 Vuelta a España plus the 1988 Tour of Britain. Now, nearly every WorldTour team relies on Sheffield-born technology to decide when to attack on a climb, where echelons might form, which rider should focus on certain stages... Basically, to shape their race strategy for the entire season.

'It's been a strange 10 years,' says Ben Lowe, founder of the phenomenon that is VeloViewer. 'But it's going well.' Clearly. I've driven up from Bristol to uncover the story behind the software that's used religiously by 17 of the 18 WorldTour teams (only Trek–Segafredo's men's teams don't subscribe to it) and learn the minutiae of course reconnaissance to add to my own performance chances. We'll see, but even if I don't turn the knowledge into application, I suspect this will be a fascinating insight into the preparation detail at the elite level.

Lowe has welcomed me into his farmhouse, which has just undergone a huge and expensive renovation, the core of which is a kitchen that's the size of a service course. More bifolds than you can count on two hands let the light pour in to reveal premium detail like the downdraft induction hob, the elegant taps and smooth flooring. 'Yes, they're from Bora–Hansgrohe and Quick-Step,' Lowe says, grinning. 'They had to be.'

It's the first inkling that while Lowe's magnificent abode is built on the fruits of his professional cycling labour, he's a fanboy at heart. Further clues are evident in every room, especially his office, where signed cycling shirts hang from the wall. We'll come back to that but for those of you not embedded in a team car or married to Strava, just what exactly is VeloViewer?

'Briefly, it's used by thousands of cyclists and runners around the world to analyse their sessions,' he says, as we ease into our interview, so much so that Lowe's enjoying the sunny rays on a sun lounger while I'm slightly raised on chair. His two dogs look equally languid on this summer Monday in June. 'But you're here for the professional use, which revolves around pre- and in-race route analysis.'

That's underplaying it. VeloViewer, or more accurately VeloViewer powered by Strava, features a WorldTour package that comprises two main parts: a race hub and a live app. Each team has its own race hub that lists all of their races for the season plus links to the details of each race and stage. Nothing ground-breaking there, you might say, but for each stage or race, the directeur sportif can add any number of customised way markers to Lowe's additions, highlighting the location of sections of the parcours that they deem important, whether it's a narrow stretch of road approaching a *petit* French village where positioning at the front is vital for the upcoming sprint or the gradient on a climb that would suit your main climber's attacking intentions. This is then displayed in the live app in the car, for adding further way markers when doing a recon or during the race to keep tabs on your team cars and the upcoming profile. Essentially, it's a high-tech roadmap that can make or break a rider's ambitions.

Team Sky popularised the marginal gains theory and garnered a reputation for their military-like precision. And it was their eye for detail that transformed the life and times for software developer Lowe.

'I wrote my first bit of coding for VeloViewer in 2012. I'm a keen cyclist myself and had just done a spin session with my then club. Afterwards, we went into the sauna at the gym and one of my mates started talking about Strava. I'd never heard of it. I was in the innovation team for a place that coded software for education and remember that the Microsoft guys were pushing us to build Windows phone apps. Anyway, I played around with Strava and noticed that there was an API...'

'A what?' dinosaur me asks. 'It stands for Application Programming Interface,' Lowe clarifies. 'You can access data from it. So, I started thinking, what is it that Strava doesn't do? It didn't show how many top-10 placings you might have had on certain ride segments, so I started with that basic model and built an app from that.'

Lowe wanted to bolster his CV so he coded and built an accompanying website, too. 'Then some guys from my club saw it and asked if they could see segments they'd ridden. It wasn't hard. You got their Strava number, coded it into VeloViewer and it would update their data every night. Then a group of Norwegians contacted me. I hadn't told anyone about it but they'd found it via a forum somewhere. They asked to be set up.'

Interest from the global amateur cycling community snowballed. Lowe added features but time was becoming squeezed. He was still working full time. His wife, Anna, was pregnant with their second child, meaning Lowe coded when Anna hit the sack at 8 p.m. He'd work until 1 a.m. every night. It wasn't sustainable: he'd soon hit the wall and, of course, Anna wouldn't be pregnant forever and there would be a new-born on the scene.

That's when Lowe decided to charge £9.99 a year, with an eye on quitting his day job to focus on VeloViewer. 'I was so nervous. I didn't have a clue about pricing strategies or anything like that. I thought I'd launch it at one in the morning, so it was a kind of soft release. A couple of minutes later I looked in my PayPal account and the first payment came in. And then a second. I stayed up for an hour just watching it, before going to bed.'

Lowe soon quit his job. By this time, VeloViewer had grown beyond recognition, proving visually and practically more usable, with one refinement in particular catching the eye of the professionals. 'I'd had 2D profiles of the routes, especially the climbs, but then remembered playing a rally video game in the 1980s that featured a 3D map. So, I worked on that via a segment in the Peak District. I'd just ridden it that weekend, so I plugged in the data from my ride and created this 3D profile with different colours depending on the gradient of that particular section. It looked very cool.

'One Tuesday night down the local pub, I got chatting to one of the lads at the club I occasionally ride with now, 7 Hills, who would often ride in the Donny Chain Gang...' The Donny Chain Gang is one of the most famous training groups in the country. It's a loose association of north-eastern riders, named after Doncaster, and made up of quality amateurs and the occasional professional. 'He mentioned that Swifty [Ben Swift, from Rotherham, who rode for Team Sky between 2010 and 2016 and is now back with them in their Ineos Grenadiers guise] said they'd been shown VeloViewer 3D profiles in their race briefings. I couldn't believe it.'

The professional seeds had been sown. Robbie Hunter of Garmin–Sharp emailed Lowe for more detail, French Eurosport used the 3D profiles and, the most flattering of all, Team Sky's Bernie Eisel started following VeloViewer on Twitter.

By 2016, Lowe had formalised an agreement for Team Sky to use VeloViewer. Back then it was just the race hub, Lowe fastidiously transforming crude and often erratic race-course GPX files into accurate maps. The live app would come from Team Sky's involvement.

'I was really encouraged by the directeurs sportifs Nico [Portal] and Dario [Cioni]. That was Team Sky in their pomp and it was the best advert I could have. I went on holiday that year and stayed with my brother, who lives just outside Chamonix. The Tour was passing by and featured a mountain time trial from Sallanches to Megève, which I think Chris Froome won [he did]. Orica [now Team BikeExchange] were staying nearby. I'd had an email from one of their DSes, Matt Wilson, who wanted to chat. Matt Hayman had seen it [VeloViewer] used in its infancy when at Sky, had moved to Orica and mentioned it to Wilson.

'Well, I met up with Wilson at the hotel, talked things through and was awestruck. Everywhere I looked there were world-class riders: Hayman, Michael Albasini, one of the Yates brothers… It was crazy. But they showed interest so I said to Sky, "I'll need to charge you now. It'll be this much if you want exclusivity" – I made up a stupid price – "or cheaper if you don't mind other teams paying for it." They chose the latter, which proved good for business.'

We remove ourselves from his Peak District garden and head inside. I want to see where the VeloViewer magic happens. Where do Ben and his team work? 'It's just me,' he replies. 'Well, I do occasionally hire a contractor but it's really just me. As for the office, it's through here.' Which is back through the kitchen, past the Alpe d'Huez illustration, to the left of his own Wattbike and next to his jump bike. It's a cycling historian's dream with cycling books galore, a picture of Lowe in action at a local hill-climbing race and, of course, those cycling tops.

'That rainbow-striped one, that's from [Annemiek] van Vleuten [it's signed, "Thanks Ben! Vleuty"]. I saw her at the Yorkshire World Championships in 2019 and asked if she had a spare jersey. She kindly gave me this one, which has a hole in it. She's actually used it a fair bit.' There's also T-shirts from Primož Roglič, the Belgian cyclo-cross team, EF–Education, Arnaud Démare … but the most treasured is the top from Team Sky. 'It's from Froome's victory at the 2017 Vuelta a España and all the riders signed it,' Lowe says. 'But it's actually Nico's gilet. He was such a lovely human being but died of a heart attack in 2020. He was only 40. He gave it to me the day before the storming day on the Finestre.'

Nico Portal touched the hearts and minds of everyone he met. A solid journeyman in his professional riding career, he excelled as a DS when Dave Brailsford gave him the opportunity to work in management on retiring at just 30 years old because of a cardiac arrhythmia. Tactical acumen married with Gallic charm were a formidable mix, and he was one of the architects of arguably the greatest stage of recent history, and one that showed off VeloViewer to its full potential.

Injury and erratic form saw Chris Froome line up for stage 19 of the 2018 Giro d'Italia over three minutes behind leader Simon Yates and struggling in fourth. Froome was aiming to wear all three Grand Tour jerseys at once after winning the 2017 Tour de France and Vuelta a España. He was nowhere near. But then a plan was hatched.

'We looked at the stage,' former head coach Tim Kerrison told former BBC journalist Tom Fordyce. 'Where Finestre, this brute of a climb, was positioned was strategically interesting. It was going to take about an hour and five minutes to ride it. You realised that if all of the top guys rode as hard as they could to the summit, they would be the only ones left. No teammates, no domestiques.

'We thought Simon was tiring. And the start of the climb has 27 hairpins. For each hairpin you decelerate into each one and have to accelerate out of it. The first four or five guys in the line are OK. When you go to 11, 12, 13, you're having to sprint out of every one. You get natural gaps. You know that if you take it on at the front, someone will pay the price at the back. Right. We will hit those hairpins as a team and hit them as hard as we can, within what Chris could maintain for an hour and a half. Simon will struggle then.'

Three big climbs peppered the last 100km of the stage: the Finestre: 18.5km long at an average 9.2% gradient and peaking at 2178m; a fast, technical descent flowed into the climb of Sestriere: 16km, the first 7km almost flat, the remainder averaging only 5%; and the ascent to the finish at Bardonecchia: 7.2km at an average 9%.

With nothing to lose, they went all in for Froome. Key was to break on the Finestre … and extend his stage lead. Solo breakaways are a rare thing in professional cycling, training by numbers levelling the playing field. For it to work, Kerrison analysed the stage on VeloViewer and calculated that Froome would need feeding at

10-minute intervals on the Finestre climb, so that he could avoid carrying the extra weight of food and fluid. So, everybody in the team – from the press officer to the security guard – was charged with delivering provisions.

It worked, Froome breaking his rivals on the Finestre and cycling to stage and, ultimately, race victory.

Lowe's far too humble to take any credit. But his software is now essential viewing in every team car and every team hotel. And mightily in-depth. He logs into his admin account and we're confronted with hundreds of races from around the world, each of which Lowe has worked his magic on, which in a reductionist way starts with ironing out those GPX files from race organisers before passing the refined version to the teams. Common GPX oversights are tunnels not being spotted and elevation gains being too high or too low due to 'spiky data'.

Organisers can occasionally be culpable of not making Lowe aware of course changes. 'I remember Milan–San Remo a couple of years ago. There was a section on the coast and the riders double back around and someone crashed on the corner. I was like, I don't remember that turn being in the route. So, I look back at the last GPX file the organiser sent me and they hadn't included it. Thankfully, that's a rare thing.'

I ask Lowe if Strava are still cool with him doing so well off ostensibly building on their base information. They are, especially after he helps smooth out any Strava navigational kinks, he says. Reliability is key with the teams fully trusting Lowe's elevation data, distance markers and way markers, meaning they can dispense with the pen and paper.

Lowe then shows off the live app by spotting team cars on an altitude camp in Tignes and recceing an upcoming race in France. He focuses on one race, a stage playing out the following day, and is fanboy personified. 'The team cars are in green,' he says excitedly. 'They're 10.3km from the finish. I click on the map and can see the average gradient, temperature, wind speed... Wind direction is important. We can see that the wind drops off from 20km/h early on to 5km/h later. If the arrow's white it's a tail or headwind, orange a crosswind and red a cross-tailwind. The start tomorrow is all red, so I'll hold the control key down and bring up Streetmap. Interesting, exposed fields. The DSes can take this information and plan their race strategy. Echelons are bound to form, which could see splits.'

And so Lowe goes on. It's fascinating stuff and every cycling nerd's dream. Riders have all this information to hand on their bike computers, the team in their cars, and Adam Blythe and his GCN team even use it for commentary.

Teams and riders continue to employ physical course reconnaissance work, of course, especially when it comes to key races or key stages. Being there in person is clearly preferred to on-screen, though more expensive and more impractical. And not always perfect. I remember talking to Matty White, Team BikeExchange's captivating DS, about course visualisation.

'That's where the race recce, morning recce and VeloViewer are all vital,' he told me. 'The problem is, you can look at the Giro or the Tour 10 days out and it won't look the same on race day. You know there'll be an Italian slapping tarmac 24 hours before their Giro stage starts! That's why sprint and climb prep are equally important. For the sprint, you have the barricades and millions of fans; for the climb, Alpe d'Huez as an example, it's a different proposition in May compared to July. God knows how many drunken fans edge close to the riders. It can make it claustrophobic.

'A perfect example's London 2012,' he continued. 'I was manager of the Australian team and knew the TT course blindfolded. I spent months out there, knew all the corners … and got there on the day and didn't expect so many people on the course. Things that I was identifying – certain houses, certain trees – it was impossible with a 10-deep crowd.' Needless to say, Australia didn't win a medal.

I'm drowning in data and stand up for air. I'm convinced – course reconnaissance is important. In fact, vital. Prepare to fail and fail to prepare, as every respectable Akela would chant. It's time to leave Lowe and his dogs and head south to start my own preparation. But then one final column of numbers grabs my attention. 'What's

VVOM,' I ask? 'It's the VeloViewer Objective Measure. Dario [Cione] asked if we could have a number of how hard the parcours is. Anna and I had a wine or two and worked out what to call it and came up with something a little like VOMiting! It's based on how hard a stage is for a GC rider and is based more on climbing than distance. I use a GC rider as while a recreational rider might ride at one pace, a GC rider might storm it at the start and finish but ease out a little in the middle. We started with a brutal stage at the Giro d'Italia and ranked that 100. Anything over that is, well, even more brutal.'

With that I suck in the oxygen, decide to be an incredibly brave boy and nervously, with trepidation, a bead of sweat and dry mouth, ask Lowe, 'The stage from Briançon to Alpe d'Huez... What's the VVOM score?' Quick as a flash and with a couple clicks, the Tour de France 2022 profile is up. 'Oooh, it's 105. That's high. But do remember that this is based on GC riders. You might race it differently.'

I have no doubt I'll race it differently; in fact, 'ride' it differently. Race is not in my vernacular. Nor will consciousness be if I think too much about that damn '105'.

───────

Ignorance is bliss. I think that's my natural state. Apparently, it's a phrase first coined by English poet Thomas Gray in his 1768 'Ode on a Distant Prospect of Eton College'. I could see where Gray was coming from. When I'd signed up to the Étape in January, I'd got so caught up in the excitement that I hadn't properly assessed the route, focusing on the 167km distance that, while no commute, was certainly doable. When I did remove my buried head from the pit of sand, I had to keep looking skywards in an effort to wrap my fatigued and increasingly threatened brain around the idea of climbing over 4700m in one day. On signing up, Alpe d'Huez had jumped out. It's iconic, has 21 hairpins and I once partied in a nightclub there called Igloo Discotheque. It's tough but, in the early days of this 'adventure', that was all I felt I needed to know. But then it became clear that Alpe d'Huez was merely the cheeseboard in a gluttonous, nay debauched, meal that'd start with the Col du Galibier followed by an indigestion-inducing main course of the Croix de Fer.

There's a reason that Briançon to Alpe d'Huez was given the moniker 'Queen Stage' for the professionals at the Tour de France, who'd race the same parcours four days later. The Galibier is Andorran in magnitude (*see* Chapter 9), measuring 23km long at an average gradient of 5.1% and topping out at 2642m. There follows a descent before the Croix de Fer, which pours scorn over the tiddler that is the Galibier by reaching out to 29km at a similar gradient of 5.2%. The one saving grace is its peak is 'just' 2067m high.

The more I stared at those figures – and the '105' that was now seemingly imprinted in luminescent form on my eyelids every time I blinked – the more I focused on something Lowe had mentioned. 'I find it interesting from a psychological perspective whether knowing what's coming up is better or not knowing is better,' he said. 'If you're broken and don't know what's coming up, is that better than being broken and knowing there's an 11% spike coming up? I guess both are demoralising in their own ways!'

Don't become a therapist, Ben.

Still, I'd done the training, recently completed my longest training ride of just under six hours, lost weight, continued to consume beetroot shots in place of alcohol, which I'd banished in the build-up to the Étape, and felt good. I'd continued with my more intense but shorter indoor sessions, the summer sun not enough temptation to override the practicality of waking and pedalling. I'd continued to attack more hills during my weekly longer rides, which had alleviated my Andorran-fuelled anxiety slightly. We'd also set a date for our house completion, found a rental that we were to move into just after the Étape, my wife was improving slowly from long Covid, our son had just taken his A-levels and everything was pointing in the right direction.

After heading north to understand the detail that goes into a WorldTour team's race strategy and tactics, I'd belatedly spent time analysing the profiles and becoming dizzy looking at gradients on VeloViewer, which is just as much available to amateurs as to the elites. The empirical overview was sorted. But to gain next-level insight, it was time to dig deep into my journalistic contacts book and seek out the anecdotal. Which is why I'm currently being stood up on Zoom. No answer. 'Five minutes,' the email comes through. Take two.

'Morning Sleeping Beauty,' I say when my Zoom partner finally appears on my screen. 'Sorry about that,' he apologises. 'Little hiccup, as I overslept. I was in Naples but now I'm back in my little flat in Tuscany. Let's shoot...'

The Tuscan narcoleptic is Andy Hampsten. Cycling fans of a certain vintage will know him well. Hampsten was the 'other' American, racing professionally between 1984 and 1996 when Greg LeMond was stealing the headlines for becoming the first non-European to win the Tour [in 1986]. For good measure, LeMond would win it again in 1989 and 1990. Hampsten actually supported LeMond during that maiden victory; both raced for the famous La Vie Claire team, before Hampsten sought his own spotlight by signing for the 7-Eleven team in 1987. It shone brightly and quickly, the Ohio-born rider becoming the first rider to win the Giro d'Italia just one year later. He now earns a living hosting bike tours.

He clearly hosts a fair few as he's a 60-year-old who looks like he could still race the Tour de France. Let's hope his memory is equally as sharp because I've tapped up Hampsten not to feel physically inferior or to talk about his time in the *maglia rosa* but to reflect, unpick and seek advice from his most memorable Tour de France moment: stage 14, Sestriere to Alpe d'Huez, Sunday, 19 July 1992.

'That was the only stage I won at the Tour,' he says. 'I was actually racing for overall that day and got into a breakaway midway through the stage. Which in hindsight looks like something I should have tried more often but it's not easy. If you're challenging for GC, you're a marked man.'

On a suffocatingly hot day in the Alps, Hampsten faced a similar parcours to me, but battled the Galibier, Croix de Fer and Alpe d'Huez after starting from Italy rather than Briançon. 'The break went on the Croix de Fer, so there were about half a dozen of us come the base of Alpe d'Huez. There's about 12km of flat from the base of Croix de

Fer to the start of Alpe d'Huez and we had several minutes' advantage over the rest.

'I recall I rode hard tempo at the front on the lower half of the climb but didn't resort to mind games. Often, you'll pretend you're strong when you're not and vice versa but we all knew we were in good condition because the break went on an uphill. And we were all good riders. [Claudio] Chiappucci and Franco Vona were the most concerning because they finished first and second the day before on a marathon stage to Sestriere [254.5km from Saint-Gervais]. There was Éric Boyer, a good French climber. And Jesús Montoya from a Spanish team [Amaya Seguros]. And Jan Nevens, I believe, a good Belgian climber.

'In the last third of the climb, I thought I'll do three very hard attacks all out. That dropped two riders. When it steepened through the village with 3km to go, I put everything on the line. It's easy on Alpe d'Huez, with the huge number of enthusiastic fans, to go too hard, to get too excited and overcook it. But my lungs, my legs, everything felt great that day and I took the win.'

Hampsten crossed the line in 5.41.58, 1.17 minutes ahead of Vona and 2.08 minutes clear of Boyer. It elevated him to third overall and he'd eventually finish fourth come Paris. Which is all wonderful for the American, his family, his supporters and his country but what I want to know is: are the Galibier, Croix de Fer and Alpe d'Huez really that tough? Cycling does have a habit of mythologising suffering. Is this real pain or an artifice forged by exuberant journos?

'Oh, it's painful alright.' Damn. 'The 21 hairpins of Alpe d'Huez are well known, which might hide the fact it's awful at the beginning. Like a lot of light climbers, I never enjoyed starting a climb hard. You want to simmer, then medium, medium high and then boiling towards the end. But it's steep at the bottom – around 10% for the first couple of kilometres. Then it taps out pretty steadily between 6 and 8%. It rises out of Huez village [around 5km from the finish] but does ease a little near the end. It's a tough end to a tough day. Just hope you don't have the day I endured there three years earlier...'

'What happened in 1989?' I asked far too impulsively. A peloton of regret is heading my way. 'Our entire team got food poisoning from this wretched little place in France that was on the border. Us riders said this place is terrible. There's a restaurant just 500m over there in Italy, let's go there. But we didn't.

'We had this frozen lasagne and it was still cold in the middle. You'd find a lot of places you stayed in were just ill-equipped. What you have is a hotel in the mountains that's been mothballed since the skiing season ended in winter. Then the Giro d'Italia or the Tour de France comes to town, so suddenly all of these little businesses are asked to open and cope with huge numbers of spectators, riders and staff.

'The place we ate in probably just served sandwiches and sold cigarettes normally, but they had to feed 20 people on the 7-Eleven team, plus media. We all got ill. I remember Eric Heiden was with us. He was a commentator working for CBS Television, I think. It was funny because he'd be in his shorts as it was so hot, but with a blazer on as he was shot from the waist up. I remember him going through his lines and he just chucks up all over the other presenter's shoes. It was a disaster.

'So that day in '89, I hadn't eaten anything all day long during the stage and was just drinking water. But I went as hard as I could because Eddy Merckx was in our car. He sponsored our team; we rode his bikes. "I'm going to watch Andy win today," he smiled. I finished 60th and came apart at the seams. I really suffered even though it didn't look like it.'

Hampsten still reached the Alpe d'Huez peak in less than five and a half hours but mental note made: no cheese the night before the Étape.

His recollections of the Galibier are mixed. Ascending, he says, isn't too bad, that 5% average a stream of lethargy compared to the shockwave of Alpe d'Huez. 'But do remember it's tricky on the descent. I remember there was always this wet corner as, even in July, there always seemed to be a snowfield dripping across the road.' Global warming might have solved that problem. 'Enjoy it, though,' Hampsten adds. 'Descending the Galibier followed by the Télégraphe on the same stretch, which amounts to around 50km, is one of the miracle descents on the planet, albeit it's actually quite tiring for that long.'

And potentially quite chilly at the top. Hampsten would often nab a newspaper off a spectator and stuff it down his top for added thermal protection at the higher, cooler climes and impending higher speeds and greater windchill. Which raises the issue of heat. A cool breath might blow over the peaks but, for the most part, the heat could very well billow ferociously in the Alps during mid-July.

'I used an alcohol-based sunscreen called Bullfrog,' Hampsten recalls. 'It's dead clear, tingles a bit but it really worked – I never got burnt. Just keep it out of your eyes. The soigneurs would also load us with wet sponges, which I'd place on the nape of my neck. You have a lot of nerves there and it's close to the brain, so really helped with cooling. Nowadays, I take a wet bandana and fold it in half to make a triangular wrap. I keep the bulk of it on the back of my neck, loose so it's not choking, and it cools nicely.'

You'll need it on the Croix de Fer, Hampsten adds, as it's tougher than the Galibier and will be tackled at the hottest part of the day. 'And pay attention again downhill. It's one of the scariest descents I've ever ridden. The first time I raced it was in 1986 and I was trying to follow a group chasing [Bernard] Hinault and [Greg] LeMond. It was 100km/h stuff and I just couldn't see where the road was going to go. So do your research.

'Look at the maps in detail,' he says, warming to the course-recce theme. He'd love VeloViewer. 'And ask around. Teammates like Sean Yates, Steve Bower and Phil Anderson were great for that. Yates especially knew every climb intimately and, if he didn't, he'd find someone in the area who did. Instead of just numbers, it was an interpretation through other riders, which was invaluable.'

As you have been Mr Andrew Hampsten and your 30-year-old physique. I've learned a lot and am toeing the line between being mentally more prepared and mentally more scared. I've trained consistently and remained injury-free but those mountains still loom very large. For Hampsten, well, he consumed cols for breakfast, lunch and dinner. It was his job, his life, his everything. His insight is appreciated and his warm spirit is contagious. If I could shrink Hampsten into an office snow-shaker, he'd doubtless provide a wonderfully motivating start to any day. But his 'interpretation' through other riders' sign-off resonated. In many ways, I'd asked Usain Bolt to help me run sub-20 seconds in the 200m. Can their empathy really reflect the reality of Everyman? They're competitors, not completers. 'I need to speak to a rider like me,' I thought. 'Someone who balances life, the universe and everything, occasionally through a mild haze of IPA. I'll call John.'

John is John Whitney, 38, and deputy editor of *Cycling Plus* magazine. He also has an encyclopaedic knowledge of road cycling. I'm actually doing John a disservice in comparing thy and I as he's conquered many mountainous sportives around the world. Which handily for me includes riding the tyrannical trio of Galibier, Croix de Fer and Alpe d'Huez in one day. There are no airs and graces with John. He'll tell me how it is. Which is why I probably put off calling him until arguably a little too late in the day. I'll just give you the 'highlights' from our chat for fear of PTSD...

THE GOOD... COL DU GALIBIER

'You're starting before 8 a.m. so it'll be cooler and you'll be riding with [16,000!] others so that'll carry you through. The Galibier's actually two climbs, really, because you're not long out of Briançon and you'll be on the Col du Lautaret. It's not a hard gradient – around 4.5–5% – but it's long. After about 13–14km, you'll fling right to the Galibier proper. This is more difficult. There are numerous switchbacks, especially when it's steeper close to the top. You can feel the wind here; that said, you'll be in a big group you can draft from. There's also a motivational boost from riding with others. Find someone to ride with – it helps. Relatively, the first climb will be easy because you're fresh, albeit bleary eyed.

'Practically, you'll be riding with two bidons. I'd be tempted to fill only one for the Galibier. Or fill both and squirt one out as you climb.

It adds weight, you'll be hydrated as it's the start and there's a drinks stop soon after the summit to refill. And take a pair of lightweight arm warmers and a lightweight gilet or jacket. You hang around in the pen for around 30 minutes at the start and it can be cold atop the Galibier. The arm warmers will also protect you from the sun later in the day.'

Note to self: ignore John's hydration advice. As a prune-like me showed at the cyclo-cross race, I need drink. And lots of it. Clothing advice? Double tick.

THE BAD... CROIX DE FER

'Prepare your mind for a long slog as nearly 30km is a long, long, long ... way to climb. You leave Saint-Jean-de-Maurienne and it's not too bad for a couple of kilometres. But then it steepens to around 10km. There's a double-edged sword after around 4km as there's a sharp descent before climbing sharply again. It's steep and you wish it wasn't there. You have the same a couple of times on Croix de Fer, which is like the Télégraphe on the Galibier. You're climbing for ages but then descend. Your body thinks it's stopped and once you climb again, your legs feel like dead weights. It's a real head fuck and you wish you could take a ski-lift. So, spin your legs a little on the descent.

'And make sure you feed when you can. Take a bento box. Some cycling snobs sneer at food-storage bags for one-day events but I'm past all that. They're really handy and can hold nutrition, tools, all sorts.'

THE UGLY... ALPE D'HUEZ

'You just won't want to be on your bike at this point no matter how well it goes; probably the worst place to be in the world right now is the bottom of Alpe d'Huez; it's debilitating and will be much more of a solo ride than an event... It's particularly grim at the start. Steep and painful. It eases a little but not enough when you're beasted. The 21 hairpins help a little as you can tick them off. And the apexes are relatively flat, especially on the outside, so it might be worth cycling longer around those. Catching people's always good for morale. But be confident that you can stay ahead. It's not good for morale to be passed again. I've ridden it as a time trial [TT] and in a sportive. The

TT was a lot easier and I rode it in less than an hour. It took double that at the end of a long, hot day in the saddle.

'I remember Greg LeMond saying that it doesn't get easier as you get fitter, you just go faster. That's bollocks. We might both be able to put out 95 per cent of our FTP, but they recover much quicker between efforts. When I've been really fit in the past, a flat switchback is enough time to recover for the next pitch. When you're not really fit, you don't recover and it's really hard to get going again. [Doing] it had been an eye-opener and felt like I was riding into hell.'

And with that, Confucius' cameo was complete. John suggested a big pre-event breakfast and bade me farewell. As (Alan) Partridge told assistant Lynn on hearing there would be no second series, 'That was a negative and right now I need two positives. One to cancel out the negative and another one so I can have a positive.'

I could either tread Lynn's path and seek salvation in a Baptist church or tap up an academic I'd interviewed several years back for a feature on fatigue and the mind. I might need the hand of God to push me up Alpe d'Huez but I chose science, setting up a one-on-one with lecturer in sports and exercise psychology at Ulster University, Noel Brick. Brick is an expert on stress management, self-talk and visualisation, and applies his knowledge beyond education, working with a number of professional athletes and teams, from Gaelic football to running and even Irish dancing. He's also an ultra-distance athlete of some repute, having completed more than 30 marathons, including the Marathon des Sables. If Brick can't impart at least two positives, no one can. Our two-wheeled therapy session begins...

Noel: What are the main challenges of the event?

Me: The heat and mountains. Visiting Andorra threw me somewhat.

Noel: Will you enjoy more time in the mountains to prepare?

Me: The event's in two weeks.

Noel: OK...

Does that mean insurmountable, Noel? As it transpires, nothing's insurmountable in Noelvana. Key to any event of this nature, he says, is keeping in the present. Of focusing on the here and now upon the

Galibier, rather than letting my mind wander to how I might feel on the Croix de Fer. 'Breaking the climb down into chunks of 5km or the next switchback is key to this because it focuses your attention on the moment. And makes these moments practical. Am I sticking to 200 watts? Am I drinking every 10 minutes? Do I need a gel? And ensure you give yourself a little clap on the back once you've reached that 5km milestone.'

This resonates. I've forever told my daughter that she spends too much time thinking and worrying rather than doing and not then having time to worry. Of course, like every self-respecting son or daughter, she doesn't listen. Worse, I'd spent so long and so much energy imparting what I thought were wonderful fatherly pearls of wisdom that I'm not used to introspection. My job as a journalist compounds this ability to look past the mirror. I've always been the hunter, not the hunted. Now it's all about me, about managing my own thoughts and actions. In the wrong hands, that could be dangerous. But Brick's advice and Irish lilt is a soothing balm. It makes sense.

'Let's go back to that Andorra visit and the worry about continuing to climb when you're already high up. I see that as an extremely positive experience. What I mean is that it prepares you for the inevitable thoughts you might have. You now know what you might be thinking during the event.

'It's about reframing your thoughts. What I advise is taking an A4 sheet of paper and having two columns. One will be what am I likely to say to myself? What will I worry about? It might be I'm 15km up the mountain, still going up and have 10km left of the Galibier, for example. Counter [in the second column] will be what will I say to myself at this point? What would be helpful? We call this, "If Then" planning. If I think this, if I worry about this, [then] what will I do? How will I respond? When we have a plan, the negative distraction becomes less of a concern.'

Brick can see I'm frozen with introspection. 'Put another way, what are the three things you take confidence from? We often detach preparation from confidence; we've done all this prep but are nervous. Anchor confidence from specific things you've done.'

And, dropping my natural guard of scepticism for a moment, I realise that there are many. Apart from a couple of short spells of missed sessions, where good old sniffles laid me low, I've stuck diligently to the training plan. The weekly long ride grew and grew to that peak I mentioned earlier of just shy of six hours, which might have bored the synapses at times but has hopefully laid an endurance foundation for what's to come. If anything, it's acclimatised my buttocks to the solid saddle. There's been the cyclo-cross experience, Tour of Flanders sportive, a midweek time trial plus hours upon hours chasing virtual riders on the Wattbike and Zwift.

I've always felt I've responded more positively to a dangling carrot (Brick) rather than a beating stick (Whitney). (OK, I'm being sensitive – Whitney's words were an honesty stick, not a beating one!) Whether that's true remains to be seen in France. But for now, living in this moment with Brick, I'm starting to grow wings, albeit ones with feathers that are receding slightly.

'I guess one of the overriding concerns of all of this is that I'm 45 years old,' I say. 'In my head, I'm 20 years younger. In my body, I'm most definitely not.'

'You've done endurance events before, right? I'm sure you were nervous before your first marathon, your first triathlon and there'll always be unknowns. But you have clear evidence of having these thoughts before and coming through it. Draw on that. And take confidence from being 45. All your life, you've been fit and active, eating well. All those things will help you now. You haven't smoked 40 or 50 a day for the last 20 years, so preparation for this event hasn't just been six months, it's been a lifetime.

'It's about reframing those age-related thoughts. You're not 20, but what experiences do they have? You're experienced at pacing, for example. Everyone storms off the start line. My strategy to deal with that is I could see these riders in five hours' time. It reassures me about my processes and not theirs, and theirs might be faulty. You can't control things like heat, altitude, distance… They're the realities of the event. But you can control your processes and strategies. This is your race, not theirs.'

Fly with me Brick, fly with me.

'Before I leave you to it, here are three things to give you a lift. Returning to chunking, when it comes to Alpe d'Huez, use those 21 hairpins to your advantage. One strategy I'd suggest is counting up to halfway, so one down, two down … and then counting down from halfway, so 10 to go, nine to go. It'll give you a lift.

'Write a reminder on your water bottles, be it something motivational, like why you're doing this, or your strategy, like 5km chunking. It's easy but powerful.

'And have a nutritional treat. This might sound crazy, but I use a lot of gels when ultra-running but I also takes Skittles with me. Every so often, I'll treat myself to one or two Skittles. It's amazing how much you look forward to the next Skittle! It reminds you of the process and part of that process is getting nutrition on board. And gels can become monotonous.

'Ultimately, everything I've been talking about is framed around something called A Theory of Challenge and Threat States in Athletes[29]. A threat state is what we talk about when we're feeling really nervous and anxious before an event. We know a threat state can impact us physiologically. It can reduce power output, blood pressure increases because blood vessels constrict, there's less oxygen flowing to your legs… Taking control [chunking], self-efficacy [confidence from what you've done] and having an approach focus [strategies and processes for the race] challenge these states. Practise them over the next couple of weeks.'

I won't let you down, Noel. By the time I arrive in France I'll have practised your techniques so much I'll be higher than the Galibier…

11

Exorcism at the Étape

T – race weekend

It's Friday, 8 July 2022. I'm at home, my Vitus squeezed and strapped into a loaned Bike Box Alan. I love Bike Box Alan because it's called Bike Box Alan. And I can see why Alan and his boxes have proved so popular, this hard-plastic number in theory protecting my bike from overzealous baggage handlers.

Two weeks today, we'll move from our home of nearly 14 years, meaning Alan's standing proud against myriad cardboard boxes, bubble wrap, brown tape stress and general irritation. And to be honest the stress and irritation are emanating from me. But domestic instability is the last thing on my mind. In any build-up to a big event, I'm inflicted with nerves, grumpiness and a short temper. Thankfully, Noel Brick's advice does elicit a mild calming effect but this Unholy Trinity remains impossible to sidestep completely because of the magnitude of the challenge: three hors catégorie climbs and nearly 170km in the midst of a European heatwave. (As an aside to alleviate the mild anxiety about my upcoming Alpine adventure, I distract myself by dipping into the Tour archives. Legend has it that mountain classification was originally calculated via a Citroën 2CV. If the old 35 horsepower car could make it up the climb in fourth gear, it was category four; third gear, category three, and so on. If it couldn't make it up the climb, it was hors catégorie. I'm unsure of the science behind that story but I really hope it's true. As you were…)

That's despite a recent repeat physiological audit, back at Silverstone, which revealed that the training and nutritional tweaks have worked. My weight has dropped to 85.5kg. That's no sub-60kg Pidcock, but this 1.88m-tall amateur is pleased. According to respected US coach Joe Friel, a 1kg loss allows you to climb a 1000m hill with a gradient of 10% around three to four seconds quicker with the same power output. Friel's calculations might not be linear but let's say they are and I apply that template to the 29,000m-long Croix de Fer, with an average gradient of around 5%. I've lost – well, not lost, worked very hard to get rid of – roughly 5kg since the start of Mosley's 24-week plan. So, in my rough pseudo-maths model, say I'm two seconds quicker per 1000m per kilogram burned. That's 10 seconds. Multiply that by 29 and that's 290 seconds or nearly five minutes saved. To be honest, when I put it like that, it makes me wonder what I have been training for!

Then again, it's all highly reductionist and I hadn't taken into account other factors like aerodynamics savings from better bike set-up and positioning (thank you Phil Burt) and arguably a better bike in the Vitus (thank you Vitus engineers). Unable to dig deep into my shallow pockets for a Vorteq wind-tunnel session, I didn't have solid data to gauge how much or how little improvement these things had brought about. But anecdotally things felt much smoother and more sustainable.

What I did have were fresh numbers, and both my VO_2 max and functional threshold power were headed in the right direction. For the former, I'd broken the 50ml/kg/min barrier with a 51. It was no Oskar Svendsen or George Bennett but it was an improvement on the original 47 and would hopefully mean sufficient oxygen delivered to my increasingly fatigued muscles in France. Arguably the biggest, and most significant, upgrade was my FTP, which had risen from 215 watts at the start to 258 watts. The majority of my sessions had been based around nudging this figure up thanks to threshold and sub-threshold efforts that gradually raised my FTP ceiling. These were the domain of the indoor Wattbike sessions – which because of my training schedule, were shorter, more intense and ticked off before breakfast.

Physiologically, things were set, apart from one thing – my ferritin levels. A week before the Étape, I'd belatedly taken another blood test with Forth Edge. The results had just arrived and all was normal, apart from the one that I really didn't want to be 'not normal'. Ferritin is a blood protein that stores iron, so its level in the blood indicates whether you have iron deficiency. Iron is essential for making red blood cells to carry oxygen around the body. Its importance cranks up further at altitude, where the air is thinner, and is why Sam Rees had waved me off from the Altitude Centre with the now prophetic words: 'Just make sure your iron levels are topped up before you go. It's a real struggle at altitude if they're not.' As much of the Étape is over 1500m, this could prove an oxygen-starved blow. I take an iron tablet. Two. And eat red meat for supper that night.

So, physiologically, I'm generally in a good place. But psychologically, I'm on edge, partly because of the trio of hors catégorie climbs ahead but arguably more so due to the challenge of just reaching the start line in the first place.

I'd already leaped over a late hurdle, namely obtaining *un certificat médical*. This is mandatory for any organised cycling event in France and is basically a document saying you're fit to race. In theory, you can get one of these from your doctor. In practice, it proved impossible. I'd been given different responses from different receptionists and had absolutely no confidence that *un certificate* would be forthcoming, especially as I'd left it until two weeks prior to the event. The clock was ticking. Thankfully, John from Chapter 10 had endured this Kafkaesque bureaucracy before and directed me to the Sports Tours International site, where I could obtain said certificate for the breezy outlay of £65. I paid my money and within a couple of days I had an official certificate from a doctor, whom I'd never met, saying I was fine to ride all day over mountains and in oppressive heat in another country. The system seemed somewhat fraudulent and rather dangerous. It was also boringly bureaucratic but unavoidable as the organisers would quite understandably cross-check things at registration.

So, certificate sorted; passport up to date; Alan packed with bike, pump and race nutrition (which I'd stored in a transparent bag with a sheet stuck to the front saying 'Nutrition' in case the French airport officials thought my energy powder contained something with a little more kick); and bags packed, which included an extra cabin bag for my helmet, clothing, shoes and pedals, which I'd removed in case my bike ended up elsewhere and I needed to hire a road bike.

There was just the small matter of transport. The plan was thus... I've included prices in case you fancy having a go at the Étape yourself. I'd fly from Bristol to Lyon Airport (£222.87 including £90 for the bike and extra for the larger cabin bag) on the Friday afternoon. I'd arrive at 7.30 p.m. and rent a car from Hertz (£245 plus £300 blocked from debit card until return. Note: you have restricted choice if you don't have a credit card). It was a three-hour drive to Briançon, which I thought would be too far late at night, so I'd booked an overnight stay in Grenoble (B&B hotel, £46) as it was about halfway between Lyon and Briançon.

I'd wake early on the Saturday and drive to Briançon to register and collect my race accoutrements (number, course profile for the top tube, etc.) before heading to Hotel Edelweiss (£78). There, I'd offload everything I needed for the race, plus a small rucksack containing toothpaste, brush and the like, as the organisers would accept small bags to shuttle to the finish area. That's because unlike many endurance events I'd done, this was a point-to-point event, not an out-and-back, meaning I'd start in one place and finish in another, in this case 80km away at Alpe d'Huez. So, unless I wanted to (hopefully) finish on the Sunday night and then ride back to Briançon to collect the car (I suspected I wouldn't be able to walk, let alone ride), I needed a car near the finish.

There will be questions at the end – stick with me.

So, after the Edelweiss crew had agreed to store my gear in their cellar as it was far too early for check-in, my plan was to drive the near two hours to Langley Hotel Le Petit Prince (£150; the area's not cheap) in Alpe d'Huez to drop off the car at their car park. Organisers ASO then laid on a shuttle bus back to Briançon. Unfortunately, I'd discovered this fact late in the day and there was no room on the bus. That meant a long online search during which I'd calculated a bus route that'd take me from Alpe d'Huez to Le Bourg-d'Oisans, which is nestled in the valley before you hit the famous climb. I'd then have to change buses again for a 90-minute trip back to Briançon.

It was a logistical labyrinth and led to a certain self-flagellation as this was a schoolboy error. Plus the costs had escalated somewhat, edging close to the £1000 mark once petrol, food and buses were taken into account. This wasn't the relatively frugal cobbled adventure of times gone by (well, Chapter 5!) and made me think I'd erred somewhat in not signing up to one of the many race packages available. As a snapshot, Ride International Tours offered entry plus a three-day stay, which included breakfast, mechanical support and transfers, for around £900. They also provided a spectator itinerary for non-cyclists, which my wife would have used if she wasn't still enduring the effects of long Covid. It didn't include flights but those were the easiest aspect to sort. In short, if you're like me and try to scrimp whenever you can, don't be short-sighted. If you're signing up to a big adventure, let an experienced company cradle you to the start line and hopefully celebrate with you at the finish line.

The thought of all this left me a nervous bundle of non-joy back in Bristol. Thankfully, my pre-race anxieties reduced with every transit box ticked. My wife had dropped me off at Bristol Airport at around 2 p.m. on the Friday. Her kiss and a hug were far more emotional than the send-off from our preoccupied children, who at 23 and 18 arguably didn't realise I'd gone. Praise be, the flight was on time and the landing into Lyon was on time. My Bike Box Alan appeared and, after a surprisingly smooth experience at the car rental, where even Alan fitted into said car (I was concerned Alan might be too wide despite double-checking online dimensions), I drove the 90 minutes to Grenoble. Granted, my affordable accommodation nestled in an industrial estate. But the bed was comfy, sleep was forthcoming and, come the Saturday morning, I was up and driving by 7.30 a.m. A leisurely drive to Briançon, accompanied by local radio, reflected an easing of the nerves. (Another aside: French law dictates that at least 40 per cent of all music played on the radio must be performed in French. My wife loves this as she loves the French language. My Devonian-meets-Bristol twang's not quite as sexy, apparently.)

I arrived at the Parc des Sports car park in Briançon at around 9.30a.m, 30 minutes before registration opened. It would prove a memorable pitstop in my no-pro journey in more ways than one. I parked up and removed my Vitus from Alan's clutches. Now, this was another of those tasks that I should have ticked off earlier but tiredness and concern over what state the bike would be in had sent my head deep into the sand. With just cause: at Lyon Airport, where cyclists poured from every nook and cranny, one poor MAMIL had opened his bike box to reveal his pride-and-joy broken and disconsolate. 'I paid £700 for this box,' he had lamented. 'But you haven't strapped it in properly, you prat,' his sympathetic mates had laughed. All the gear, no jolly idea. Yet much mirthful material for his friends to bring up forever more.

Now, at the start village and registration, it was time to pluck my massive cranium from the grains and check the state of my training partner, confidant and dream-killer/maker (I'd know which one to delete very soon). There was no other choice, this was a Pandora's Box that had to be opened. But what evil would lie within? Unlike the steed of the broken-airport-biker, it seemed to be in one piece. I reattached the wheels, raised the seatpost to the dimensions set out by the Cornishman in Chapter 2, mounted and tentatively gave it a swift spin. 'I don't believe it,' I thought. 'It's bloody working. Let's just shift gears and I'm all good…'

I wasn't all good. The electric groupset that I'd become so attached to, so impressed by the smooth, slick shifts and the boys-toys whirring with each button press, had become upset in transit. The whirring had been muted and the shifts, well, simply weren't shifting. The gears weren't working. I pressed and pressed in increasing desperation, resembling a hairier version of Basil Fawlty and his car-whacking stick, but nothing, nada, nowt. I'd opened the lid on Pandora's Box and the curse was immediate.

As the morning sun rose, so did the ambient temperature and so did my stress levels. 'OK, Jimbo,' I muttered to myself, 'do not panic.'

Breathe and think. This is rectifiable. And it is. Shimano, who made my groupset, are providing mechanical support to all entrants in the start village. Simply queue, let them work their magic and all will be fine with the world. This will work. Alternatively, I could remove the seatpost, wave it around in the Alpine air in a desperate manner to kick-start it, or reattach the battery within and see if that works. And by some luck of the cycling gods, the latter bloody did the trick. A connection point must have been lost between Bristol and Briançon and now we were reconnected. I could not believe it. À *la* an IT technician rescuing your computer by switching it off and on, I'd cut my cortisol levels by the simplest of remedies. Granted, I'd never seen a groupset repaired by waving the seatpost in the air like an airport marshal in any bike-maintenance book but it had done the job.

A smile of contentment spread over *ma visage rouge* and I could finally relax. My bike was working, I was working (not efficiently, clearly, but I was in one piece) and I could actually enjoy this moment, a moment that had seemed so far away deep in that cyclo-cross quagmire back in January. Yes, pain awaited the following day but enjoy this, I said to myself. Now that my bike had finally passed its pre-race MOT, I removed the front wheel so that bike and wheel could fit in the car, to save the minor faff of squeezing it back into Alan. I'd then drop it off at the hotel, drive to Alpe d'Huez, bus it back, sleep and ride to Alpe d'Huez. Easy.

By now, registration was open. And oh my, what a magnificent atmosphere. A huge gantry welcomed me and 16,000 other riders to L'Étape du Tour's start village, set against a stunning mountainous backdrop. The aim of this journey had been to rub shoulders with the professionals and see if any of their wisdom would inspire me to the finish line. In the here and now, that all changed. It was about me and my fellow recreational cyclists. Riders of all ages, of all nationalities, looking tanned and athletic, milled around the start village, looking at the latest gear from bike manufacturers, wheel manufacturers and training-tool manufacturers. The sun glistened on carbon and credit cards. We were a band of brothers and sisters. Each had followed their own journey to Briançon and each had a story to tell. I just had the privilege to tell my story in print in all good bookstores! Tomorrow would be the final chapter.

After a lap of the start village, I registered and made my way back to the car with my race number in hand. This was L'Étape du Tour 2022 and I was officially in it. With that, I drove out of the car park. By now, the start village and surrounding areas – more precisely, the roads – were packed with cyclists either signing on or heading off. Finally, the queues relented and I could shift out of first gear. I was on my way. I turned up the volume on the radio and threw a wry – even smug – grin at the rear view mirror. This was happening.

I checked the rear view mirror once more, this time for travel safety purposes, and noted my Vitus and Bike Box Alan. As I should, as I packed them. What I didn't notice was my front wheel. I looked to the passenger seat, for no other reason than an unfolding desperation of incompetence. All that lay there was an empty bottle of Evian and a Malt Loaf wrapper. 'Please God, no,' I thought. 'I haven't.' I had. On packing my bike into the car after groupset-gate, I'd removed the front wheel to squeeze the bike in and forgotten to squeeze said front wheel in as well as said bike. 'I cannot believe this is happening,' I thought in more parochial language. 'I must have left the wheel leaning against the car.'

Un imbécile. I turn around to face a long queue and a whirlwind of distress. Again, breathe easy. I'm sure the wheel will be on the floor at the spot where I drove off. Or guarded over by a diligent marshal. Or spotted by some kind *gendarme* and taken to lost property. 'It will be fine.'

It wasn't.

A car occupied the spot where I'd packed up the car with a grin of accomplishment after delivering my electronic groupset CPR. I spoke to the nearby stewards in panicked pidgin English about only possessing one wheel. 'No, nothing is lost in translation. I have been this idiotic.' Their looks of confusion were matched by collective '*nons*'. I visited lost property. Still no luck. The front wheel had rolled off to who knows where. What the hell would I do? A DNS (Did Not

Start) wasn't an option. I could not let all those months of training roll off down the mountain. But what were the options? Could I unicycle 170km to Alpe d'Huez? It'd certainly add a unique strand to this cautionary tale.

Then, with thoughts spiralling out of control, along with perspiration under the 30°C skies, I spotted the gazebo under which mechanics worked on hire bikes. 'Can you hire a front wheel only?' 'You want just the one wheel?' I didn't go into the detail why but yes, I did. 'We only hire out bikes.' Fair. Hiring out a bike with rear wheel only would have been even more random than hiring out the front wheel.

Around £200 later, I'd agreed to hire a front wheel. 'But the deposit is €1,000.' Which I didn't have in my account as we'd just laid out a wedge of cash for removal and storage. I phone the one person I know who I knew would have the money, understands my nuances and has online banking: my sister.

'How's it going,' Lou asked? 'Interesting...' I replied.

To cut this long story slightly shorter, my big sis agreed to a short-term loan. Finally, after much paperwork, I hired the wheel. The mechanics would collect the wheel at the Alpe d'Huez finish line, which looked optimistic at this precise moment. Stress had burned through a day's worth of energy that I'd preferred to have expended the following day, when I knew I'd run roughshod through 7,000 calories or more. Still, the bike and its overpriced front wheel worked and I'd now deposited both at Hotel Edelweiss, alongside my race attire and nutrition.

'So, all good at last?' you might think. 'Let's return to the race action, please.' Unfortunately, there were further logistical hurdles to leap over. Or collapse through. I'd haemorrhaged time sorting out my nonsense and so there was no way I'd be able to drive to Alpe d'Huez in time to then catch the last bus to Le Bourg-d'Oisans and another bus back to Briançon. It was all a little too much, so I reverted to my head-burying days and decided to park the car in Le Bourg-d'Oisans at the base of the final mountain. I'd worry about how to collect it from the hotel in Alpe d'Huez on the Monday morning. 'I could always walk the 14km after a day of torture,' I joked to myself...

Come Saturday evening, after a long afternoon drive followed by an even longer, hot, sweaty, uncomfortable bus ride back, my mood lifts. After the day of days, everything is finally in place. OK, there remained nearly 170km and 5000m of climbing ahead tomorrow in what would be a blisteringly hot day in the Alps, but right here, right now, I'm finally back in Briançon, my bike's ready, my kit's laid out, I've attached my race number (7884) to the bike and my top, my nutrition's got through customs and I'm ready to go. Just reaching this point – both on the journey as a whole and on this 'memorable' day, in particular – is a weight off my shoulders, which is clearly a good thing with the Galibier on the menu first thing.

Talking menu, the last box to tick was the general nutrition one. Once again, I'd eaten badly on race weekend, the trials and tribulations of transit leaving me eating rubbish sandwiches and snacks on the fly. I'd hydrated well, though, with a bottle of Evian forever by my side. I decide I couldn't screw up another pre-race evening without a hot meal so, after collecting breakfast supplies in the form of bread, jam and bananas, I order a pizza. Yes, I know once again this is far from textbook but my rationale is that the dough's overflowing with carbohydrates, even if they've been processed to within an inch of their lives. I kept it simple – tomato, cheese, olives and rocket. Olives contain good fats and, after interviewing Andy Jones, or Mr Beetroot, at Toby's fuelling fest, I knew rocket contains nitrates. I might need to eat an allotment's worth to enjoy blood flow-easing benefits, but still.

Pizza ordered, a motivational call from my wife done, pizza collected and I'm walking back to Hotel Edelweiss (which, sadly, only served breakfast to the minor disappointment of myself and other riders kipping here). It's all coming together, albeit the comfortable room (nice bed, decal, loo...) is actually rather uncomfortable as there's no air conditioning. Still, it's not the end of the world, though that unsettled feeling's making me a little paranoid. My stomach feels slightly bloated and has ever so slowly ballooned throughout the day. I put it down to nerves and possibly overhydrating on water.

The pizza acts as a distraction when I nearly break a molar – what sadist would not use pitted olives! – but it's not that appealing. I like *fromage* as much as the next turophile but this is drenched in the stuff. I eat one slice, struggle through the second and call it a day. This is carbo-loading of the most pitiful order but I'm sure a good sleep, a good breakfast and a good race-day nutrition strategy will compensate.

I lie on the bed. Or roasting tray. *Sans* sheets, I toss, turn and then visit the toilet. The bloating is bordering on painful. This isn't good. I won't delve into the detail but let's just say there was a jet-wash feel about proceedings, and so begins an evening of relaying between the loo and the furnace of a mattress. This rolls on deep into the small hours until just as the seas had calmed and I'd started to drift, the alarm goes off.

It's 5.30 a.m. This is the time when in my head I'd tuck into my bread and jam, chow down on a banana, drink an Americano – maybe two – slip into my bike apparel and roll down to the starting pen, from where I'd show the world that with consistent, progressive training, a good nutrition plan, a few high-tech tools, oodles of advice from pros and experts and a dollop of motivation, cycling's mythical mountain range could be conquered. Instead, I'm looking in the mirror at a perspiring ghost who still has a slight discomfort in the pit of his stomach. And it's not long before that ghost is looking at the ceramic u-bend as the limited slices of pizza with maximum amount of cheese make a reappearance. This becomes a projectile procession as five times the *fromage* of fate flows. It's unpleasant and I'm just glad my wife's not here to witness this Étape Exorcism.

Then again, I wish she was. I feel empty, a shell, emotionally in an abyss that I know my wife would lift me out of. She has a beautiful soul and is forever raising the spirits. If that comes at the expense of being meticulous about the 'mundane' – mortgage, electricity, council tax... – then so be it. The energy's been sucked out of me, my prep is in ruins and I contemplate withdrawal. I contemplate calling my wife but it's not even 5 a.m. in the UK and this beautiful soul isn't always quite as beautiful when she's lacking sleep.

I look back to the mirror. What had I done? I'd been told not to have cheese the night before the race. Andy Hampsten had also been undone by a frozen block of the stuff. Then again, that bloating began before pizza-gate. Maybe the cheese was simply the last straw.

The bike fit, the cyclo-cross, Flanders, the long Sunday rides and midweek morning efforts. Week after week. All wasted. The Étape had shadowed – at times, weighed down – every event since the year's start, from Portugal with my son to Kempo's stag-do in San Sebastián, his wedding plus countless occasions in-between. All wonderful moments but tarnished slightly by the looming mountains ahead. I'd begun to feel what elite athletes must feel when their Olympic dreams are shattered through injury. And they'd train for four years, or their whole lives, not six months. It must be devastating. At which point I begin to get my shit together.

I tell myself, 'You can stand, you can breathe, your stomach's empty. Yes, it's left a mild pain and a hint of nausea remains but the bloating's gone.' And as a positive, the evacuation has left me feeling the lightest I'd felt in years.

With nothing to lose apart from what's left of my diminishing dignity, I dress. Santini bib shorts. On. Pinnacle cycle top. On. Pair of free socks given away with the Tour de France guide I'd just edited. On. ROKA sunglasses, Rapha helmet, Van Rysel bike shoes. On, on, on. I pack a scrunched-up lightweight jacket into my rear pocket in a surprising act of optimism, in case I actually reach the peak of Galibier and need warmth for the descent. Finally, it's about arming myself with nutrition.

I planned to consume around 60–90 grams of carbohydrate an hour from various sources. I'd have two bottles, one of which was a 1000mg sodium drink from Precision Fuel & Hydration. The other would be Maurten 160. The latter is Kipchoge's drink of choice and includes hydrogel that reportedly makes digestion easier. I'd tried the 320, which is double the carbohydrate, in the cooler climes of the UK. It had worked well but I'd been warned about taking in so many calories in the heat, so I'd gone for its smaller sibling. I also packed a variety of gels and planned to stop at the four feed stations, positioned at kilometres 50, 82, 108 and 150. There, my nutrition plan could arguably unravel as I'd fill my boots with bars and cake. Or the old me would. The 'trained' me would nab a few solid morsels but stick to the carbs per hour plan. That was the theory. As it stood, all I'd managed to keep down so far was a Beet It shot. If that were to make an alarmingly reddish reappearance in the race, I'd expect to be airlifted to the nearest hospital.

Dressed and ready, I mount my bike and ride downhill to the start. It's around 6.50am. My wave's off at 7.52 a.m. with the first wave off at 7 a.m. Despite the planning, I don't have a clear set finish time in mind. I'd calculated that I'd need at least two hours on each mountain, if not more. Since much of what lies in-between is descending, I'd decided to be delighted with anything around nine hours. If that somehow edged nearer eight, I'd be knocking on the Ineos Grenadiers' door. Ultimately, finishing is the main goal, which is not a given, certainly in my current state. There's also a strict cut-off time at various points around the parcours. Fail to hit certain times and you're swept up by the broom wagon. Which at that moment on the start line seemed likely if things didn't improve.

I wait in the start pen with hundreds of others. Finally, after an eternity – no more than 30 minutes! – I was off, high-fiving Didi the Devil, aka 70-year-old Dieter Senft, who has donned a red devil costume and brandished a trident at the Tour since 1993.

Along with my cycling brethren, we're near enough straight on to the first climb of the ride, the Col du Lautaret, which would flow on to the Galibier. This is where I had two plans. The first involved sticking at around 180 to 200 watts. The second involved taking one gel for the first hour and seeing if it would stay down. There would be no solids and for now I would avoid the Maurten and just sip on electrolytes.

It seemed to be doing the job. That nauseous feeling dissipated with every kilometre that passed. I hadn't got any Imodium to hand, so I was heavily racing on spirit alone, but I was surviving, if most definitely not thriving. Still, that haunting fellow who had nearly cried in the mirror 90 minutes before had thankfully deserted me.

The heat helped, in so much that it wasn't that bad so early in the day. As John (Whitney) had predicted, riding in a large group helped, too. I latched on to a collective going at a similar pace and on we climbed. Then, after 1 hour and 53 minutes and 51 seconds, the Galibier had been conquered. OK, not conquered but surmounted. I'd later hear tales of swathes of riders being swept up by the broom wagon, failing to make the first cut-off by the time the Galibier's brutal peak was reached. Dodgy tum or no dodgy tum, this was a brute of a challenge.

And it hadn't been too bad. As Brick advised, I gave myself a metaphorical pat on the back. It seemed that the relatively regular climbs out of Bath to Lansdown had paid off. For now. The only section that had begun to burn a bit came around 5km from the peak, where the gradient averaged 8% for a couple of kilometres. Historically, I'd been fine with long and shallow, but short and sharp was a different matter. How I would cope with the long and sharp pitches ahead, plus my general state of being, would dictate if dreams were to be made or nightmares begun.

I stopped to put on my jacket. By now it was around 10.30 a.m. It wasn't really cold but doing so did provide me with an excuse to stop. I also took my first swig of Maurten. I'd written the words, 'Every turn of the wheel' on the bottle, inspired by Brick and Philosopher Kempo, who had both that morning very kindly texted me messages of support.

Then it was on to the descent, which would be nothing like anything I'd experienced before. It would cover 50km before levelling at Saint-Jean-Michel-de-Maurienne. Andy Hampsten had called it one of the great descents of the world. He has a far more extensive palmarès for downhill comparison, but it certainly proved the most exhilarating of my life. Weaving around the stunning backdrop of the Alps reminded me that at its heart, this challenge should be fun. Self-flagellation and many moments of frustration in resisting temptation had clouded that at times but on the descent of the Galibier, I remembered. Even the 5km ascent of the Télégraphe didn't temper this moment of joy as I got talking with fellow Étape challenger Cillian Kelly of YouTube channel Global Cycling Network.

The Irishman's journey had been similar to mine, trying to complete a big bike challenge without (fully) sacrificing family and friends. We rode together for around 15 minutes. He was amusing company and a very useful distraction from the brief ascent.

For one of the few times that day, I accelerated, bade Kelly farewell, adopted the drops position I'd worked on during the time trial and continued down to Saint-Jean ... and the next feed station. I wasn't feeling too bad and was encouraged by a text from my wife, who informed me I was ahead of former Formula One world champion Damon Hill. She'd been tracking me via my computer-chipped race number on the Étape website and was delighted I'd led the motor-racing legend. Yes, he's 16 years older than me at 61, but that didn't prevent another metaphorical back-patting moment.

That was the last time I patted myself on the back all day.

From here, it was straight on to the 29km-long Croix de Fer; and everything changed. A couple of gentle kilometres sheered up to a gradient of 7.9% and then 9.8%.

As the gradient rose, so did the midday sun. Respite was on the cards after 4km with a 2km descent but there was a definite dismal realisation throughout the descent that what goes down must go up. And keep on going up. In devastating fashion. Between kilometres 6 and 12, the course profile was shown as black on the map. This means bad. And it was, oscillating between gradients of 9% and over 10%. To put that in context, back in Bristol, my regular 'mountains' of Lansdown Hill and Cheddar Gorge averaged 6.8% and 4.7%, respectively, but that was for just 3km and 3.5km. They maxed out at 12.6% and 12.2% but for the briefest of moments. This was a different league. In fact, many different leagues. The Premier versus Conference. Goliath versus David...

The temperature was now well into the 30s. And I'd started to drink like a fish, always a sign of increasing desperation. I wasn't the only one. The relatively genial atmosphere atop the Galibier had been replaced by the silence of suffering. Riders began to drop to the side, for rest and to gather together their thoughts. This collective event had very much become about the individual. This was the biggest test so far. Could new depths be plumbed in an effort to reach new heights? To reach the peak of Croix de Fer?

For rider 7884 (aka me), the answer was yes. Just. But psychologically and physically, this was a new race. Thankfully, between kilometres 15 and 23, the gradient eased before rearing its ugly, steep head again near the top. This is where the first cracks appeared; in other words, I eased over to the side, off my Vitus, took a big swig of drink and walked. This was becoming a theme. In Keynsham, in Flanders, steep sections had proved to be my nemesis. In both, they were just about manageable. Here, with Alpe d'Huez to come and its average gradient of 8.1% over 13.8km, plus an increasing heat-, mountain- and sickness-derived fatigue, I was shrinking and shrivelling. Literally and metaphorically.

For good measure, the hot spot in my right foot that had been eased by Burt's good work – and insoles – reappeared with a vengeance. The pain grew so fierce that I dropped a couple of paracetamol. There was little respite on the long descent, my hazy mind meaning my fingers were either squeezing, or ready to squeeze, the brakes. By this stage, after eight hours in the saddle, I didn't trust myself or my cognition skills.

Finally, there was a level run-in to Le Bourg-d'Oisans. By now, I was parched. I'd exhausted my drinks supplies and there was still 10km to the final feed station. Then, like a Siren, a cafe appeared on the horizon. Any ambitions of finishing within 10 hours had long gone. Now it was all about completion and narrowly avoiding the broom wagon. In my fuzzy and fatigued head, the rules weren't clear about when I'd be swept up. But I roughly knew that under 12 hours and I should be OK; over 12 hours and, well, I couldn't contemplate that. The only thing I could contemplate was to stop and order the most satisfying bottle of cool Coca-Cola I'd ever drunk. Yes, cyclists were passing me in their droves but I didn't care one iota, especially as the staggered start meant I had no idea where I was in the overall narrative of the event. All I knew and all I cared about it was that it revived me. At least until the next fuelling stop, where I filled up on peaches, Jelly Babies, water, pears…

Weighed down but fuelled up, it was time for Alpe d'Huez, the most iconic climb in cycling. Ahead were 21 hairpins, each one ready to slash my chances of reaching the finish line. But I knew how to use them to my advantage, chunking each to ease my suffering and edge me towards immortality. Or something like that.

By now, I'd been on – and off – the bike for nearly nine and a half hours, the longest I'd ever been clamped to a saddle in one day. John had told me that at this stage, the last place I'd want to be was on my bike. He was right. Chapeau to bike-fitter Burt as, despite the duration, my buttocks remained free from saddle sores. But the rest of me – my legs, body and mind – were heavy and vacant. Which is why I adopted what's called a 'walking strategy' from the very beginning of the Alpe d'Huez. John had been right again – it's a nightmare from the start, averaging a gradient of over 10% for the first couple of kilometres before nudging down to around 9%. It would remain this steep until around the 11km mark.

So it was that I clip-clopped my cleated feet slowly up Alpe d'Huez. I wasn't the only one, soon hooking up with a chap from Essex called Sachin. Other riders stretched out on the sweltering concrete blocks that lined the route. This was brutal.

Thankfully, Sachin kept me sane, our occasional chat as we walked a welcome distraction from emptiness, a sore foot and dwindling hope. Not that long before, I had been confident of finishing and waving goodbye to the wagon. Now, with my speed stalling, I calculated the wagon must be close. Too close for comfort.

My head was down and when I looked up, Sachin had accelerated. More accurately, I'd decelerated. That's adding a false sense of speed as we were both still walking. Then everything began to cramp. I was in a hole. My wife and Kempo, both watching my glacial progress online on the Étape website, phoned through their support. It was a touching gesture at a time when I was fighting myself in my very hot, lonely and brutal world. I struggled to speak and just kept whispering, 'It's so hard.'

Further support came from a corner packed with Norwegians setting up for the professional efforts four days later. 'Get to the finish line, dude,' shouted a Scandinavian. 'No matter what it takes.' The positivity started to break through and recalibrated my mindset. 'It's about reaching that finish line,' I told myself. Over and over. 'And keep eating those succulent peaches.'

Further relief came via a family who were hosing down riders outside their roadside chalet. Then, with 3km to go and the sun finally losing its ferocity, Huez relented, eased its gradient to 5% and I could ride again. This wasn't an easy task, not because of the flames of fatigue that had swept over me, nor because of the pain emanating from my foot, but because I'd walked for so long that my cleats had literally ground down. Connection with the pedals was lost. It mattered not.

The psychological arc that Mark Beaumont had talked about was coming true. I'd endured misery for much of the day but with the finish line close, my mood and speed perked up. I balanced my shoes on the pedals and for the first time in around seven hours I felt no pain, even unleashing a sprint of sorts to the line. I'd done it. I'd kept the broom wagon at bay and earned my beast of an Étape medal.

I crossed the line in 11 hours and 58 minutes, way behind my ambitions and even further behind the men's winner Stefan Kirchmair, who won in a frankly ridiculous 5 hours and 17 minutes. Flávia Oliveira triumphed in the women's race in an equally ridiculous 6.5 hours. But I'd made it, along with 8450 other riders from the 16,000 who had started. Sadly, Damon Hill was one of those who didn't make the cut-off. But chapeau to Devereux – yes, that's Damon's magnificent middle name alongside his passed father's more prosaic 'Graham' – for even attempting L'Étape as the average age of 2022's cohort came in at 44 with the same number (in percentage terms) of first-timers. But Cillian Kelly of GCN fame made it; in fact, I'm sure I saw his derrière pass me near the peak of Alpe d'Huez!

It had taken me a cleat-grinding 2 hours 32 minutes and 15 seconds to ascend Alpe d'Huez. In 1997, Marco Pantani had stormed up there in a record 37 minutes and 35 seconds, a mere 1 hour 54 minutes and 40 seconds ahead of me. Pantani's time happened in the pharmaceutical age, but I could have consumed the A to Z of illegal drugs and there's no way I'd have come within a whisker – or an hour – of The Pirate.

But by now I didn't care. TrainingPeaks told me that I'd burned through 7100 calories from an average 140bpm that maxed out – many times – at 170bpm. But I didn't need the data to tell me what I knew. This had been a day of suffering like no other and I'd come through it. Just. Everyman had escaped the broom wagon but was clearly no match for the elites…

———

'Pidcock's like poetry in motion on the descent of the Galibier. He's like Messi when he sees a pass no one else sees.'
Rob Kemp, GCN and Eurosport commentator

Thursday, 14 July 2022. Bastille Day. Four days after my ordeal on the Étape and 233 years since revolutionary insurgents stormed and seized control of the medieval armoury, fortress and political prison known as the Bastille, the institution that represented royal authority and King Louis XVI's abuse of power. The French Revolution had begun. But on this sweltering Thursday in July, the monarchy had returned in the form of the 2022 Tour de France's Queen Stage, so called because it's designed to be the hardest, most demanding stage of the race.

The pros have completed 11 days of racing and had two rest days. Stage one's 13.2km time trial took place in Copenhagen, Denmark, against the backdrop of huge crowds and incessant rain, and it was Quick-Step's Yves Lampaert who upset the odds by winning. 'I'm just a farmer's son from Belgium,' an emotional Lampaert said after the stage. A farmer's son, that is, who stormed around Denmark on a 10-grand-plus Specialized S-Works Shiv TT carbon number, fitted with a Roval front wheel (around a grand) and a 321 disc wheel (over £1500) plus an electronic groupset. Lampaert did, however, refrain from wearing Specialized's much-derided TT5 time trial helmet, whose bulbous design incorporated, as *Cycling Weekly*'s Simon Smythe put it, 'a Gregory Porter-esque built-in balaclava', or head sock. Lampaert said he hadn't had a chance to try it rather than its absence being due to sartorial criticism.

Ineos Grenadiers grabbed the headlines for all the wrong reasons. Pre-stage favourite and current time trial world champion Filippo

Ganna saw the rain wipe out any marginal gains in fourth while Geraint Thomas finished down in 18th, undoing all the good and expensive work in the wind-tunnel by forgetting to remove his pre-race gilet.

By Bastille Day, all that was forgotten as the Welshman stood in fourth on the GC, just under two and a half minutes behind leader Jonas Vingegaard. Jumbo–Visma's Vingegaard had leapfrogged two-time Tadej Pogačar after winning the 11th stage from Albertville to Col du Granon, which many labelled a stage for the ages. Vingegaard and Primož Roglič repeatedly accelerated from the solitary Pogačar, who finally cracked and showed he's human. Death by a thousand attacks.

With Adam Yates in sixth and Tom Pidcock in 11th, Ineos Grenadiers could take comfort from a solid team effort. Which arguably highlighted how much their stock had dropped. After winning seven of the eight editions of the world's biggest cycle race between 2012 and 2019, now they were fighting for a podium spot. Consistency of the collective is to be admired but the expensively assembled British team needed a protagonist to remind the world of their worth.

They had form here, Thomas the last winner atop Alpe d'Huez in 2018. But a repeat looked unlikely with the 36-year-old still on the GC radar of Vingegaard and Pogačar upfront. In fact, it was their former leader and four-time Tour winner, Chris Froome, who had the spectators and commentators in raptures early on as he counter-attacked on the Galibier in an effort to reel in the early breakaway. Froome's life, let alone career, hung in the balance in 2019 after a crash on a morning recce at the Critérium du Dauphiné. Multiple fractures and a significant loss of blood later, it was a miracle he recovered to ride a bike at all, let alone be competitive. But here, against the heat and haze of the Galibier, the now Israel–Premier Tech rider showed up at the sharp end of a race for the first time in three years.

If Froome signalled his intent on the ascent of the Galibier, Pidcock's objectives were of pyrotechnic proportions on the way down. The skill of descending is often an afterthought with the grit, determination and suffering on the climbs tapping into a writer's sense of the visceral. That changes when the downhill is executed with the dexterity and fluidity of Pidcock on Bastille Day.

It was a masterclass and, by the base of the Galibier, he'd not only caught Froome but the breakaway, too. I recommend heading to YouTube and watching Pidcock's technique, again and again and again. Attacking a right-hander, it's man and machine at 45 degrees, left leg straight, right knee out, right elbow down and then he's out of the saddle, accelerating as he exits. He then mirrors that technique for a left-hander. It's metronomic and as if he's on a Scalextric on one of those rare days as a youngster when no matter how haphazardly you pulled the trigger, your car remained on track.

But this is no accident. As Kemp enthused, 'You can train to go uphill, downhill you need to grow up on a bike.' Froome echoed those sentiments afterwards: 'Pidcock was flying on the descents today. I think that his bike handling and off-road riding probably came in handy today … there were a few points where I backed off the wheel a bit because he was definitely pushing the limits.' Pidcock himself commented, 'I grew up riding my bike. I rode to school every day. I always took a detour through the woods. You know, drifting through the woods in the mud. I'd come home and my uniform was all dirty. I guess I've just become very used to riding a bike and handling it in situations where it's on the limit of control. I've a very good understanding of my bike as well. The tyre grip and everything like that. I guess it kind of comes a bit naturally.'

But Nick Craig, cyclo-cross legend, summed up Pidcock's brilliance best many months ago in the fields of Ardingly. 'I remember one cyclo-cross race years ago before Charlie passed. It's a corner I know well. It's really fast and was really slippery. Approach that corner too fast and you'll end up on your arse. I watched Tom approach the corner and he was riding way too quick. I said to [my son] Charlie, watch what happens here. Tom knew he was going too fast, so he intentionally lost both wheels sideways, unclipped his left foot – it was a left-hand corner – hit the floor and kicked himself back up again. He knew he was going too fast but he didn't care because when it goes wrong, he'd just kick himself back up again! I was like Jesus, I haven't seen that before.'

The only thing hitting the floor on Bastille Day were the jaws of rivals, spectators and commentators alike as Pidcock reached his maximum speed on the descent of the Croix de Fer, breaking the three-figure barrier at 100.8km/h. Pidcock said afterwards that he'd never hit the ton before.

Maybe it was the Yorkshireman's effort at cooling, seeking greater breeze at higher speeds. Wet sponges and tights packed with ice were the order of the day with Pidcock's post-ride data showing a maximum temperature of 42°C, though there was a degree of respite offered from riding for much of the day above 1500m, which came in at a relatively arctic 33°C.

Still, as Alpe d'Huez loomed into view, Pidcock had much to do. As the crowds expanded at the bottom of the 13.8km climb, Pidcock headed a leading quintet comprising Froome, Louis Meintjes (Intermarché–Wanty–Gobert Matériaux), Giulio Ciccone (Trek–Segafredo) and Nelson Powless (EF Education–EasyPost).

Two Covid-interrupted Tours had seemingly brought out more spectators than ever as Pidcock squeezed through. He broke early on Alpe d'Huez, holding a healthy lead by corner number seven, aka Dutch Corner. 'Welcome to orange hell, Tom Pidcock,' commentated Ned Boulting on ITV. 'Will it inspire him or intimidate him? It is a wall of noise.'

The fearless Pidcock chose the former, winning the Queen Stage of Briançon to Alpe d'Huez in 4.55.24. 'On Bastille Day,' Boulting enthused, 'fireworks on the Alpe and a star is born. A ride of pure brilliance.' Meintjes would take second 48 seconds later with Froome a fine third 2.06 minutes behind.

At 22, Pidcock had become the youngest stage winner atop Alpe d'Huez and cemented his burgeoning reputation among the hundreds of thousands of beer-drinking, Beefeater-wearing, Devil-chasing spectators. Strava revealed that over the course of just under five hours, the Ineos Grenadier rider averaged 32.8km/h. Power and heart rate data were concealed though his team did let us know that his average cadence came in at 88rpm.

Pidcock averaged 20.4km/h up Alpe d'Huez, which was plenty to hold off Meintjes and Froome, though Jumbo–Visma's Sepp Kuss, wingman to Vingegaard, was KOM for the day at 40.08mins, 10 seconds ahead of Romain Bardet. Bob Jungels, I'd like to think inspired by our chat a few months prior in the build-up to Flanders, was the third fastest, on Strava at least, thanks to a 42.42-minute effort with Pidcock at 43 minutes dead.

The fastest times recorded on Alpe d'Huez are 37.35 minutes and 37.36 minutes by Marco Pantani and Lance Armstrong in 1997 and 2004, respectively. Both doped. As mentioned before, you'd be naive to think cycling's completely free from doping but the times reflect this hope.

'It's made my Tour de France, that,' Pidcock reflected with a hint of Yorkshire at the post-stage press conference. 'If I get dropped every day from now on, I don't care. Stage win, my first Tour, it's not bad.

'The idea was to get in the break. I lost enough time yesterday to be given freedom [to attack]. Think if I'd pushed it on the climb on the Galibier, I don't think I'd have got away, but on the descent, well, Jumbo didn't want to risk chasing me. The gap was small enough to bridge across. Worked perfect in the end, actually.' Pidcock was then asked what it meant to a rider who'd already won Olympic gold? 'That was unreal. When you're literally slaloming through people's flags, fists and god knows what else, you won't experience that anywhere else apart from Alpe d'Huez at the Tour de France.'

Thomas Pidcock MBE would go on to finish 17th overall at his debut Tour de France. The youngster's surely a GC contender of the very near future, if not in 2023. At 1.7m and just 58kg, he's a world-class climber. He can descend, we know that, and despite that featherweight anatomy, he packs an absolute power punch in the time trial. He also possesses a confidence born from racing off-road and from working with what remains, despite their relative Tour drought, one of the strongest teams in the world. He has everything. But ultimately, he hadn't proved that he can cope with 12 hours of brutality in just one day. I had, so maybe Pidcock's the Everyman and I'm Superman…

12

The Debrief

T+ one day

It's 7.30 a.m. on Monday, 11 July 2022. I'd slept well in a hotel room designed for skiing groups. Hence, the four beds and one bunk bed for this solitary rider. Overkill but available. The night before, I'd planned to check out the post-event vibe in the nearby restaurants and bars, but fatigue had wrestled me to the ground, so I ended up ordering a takeaway beef burger and can of lager, both of which I hardly touched. Before I knew it, the sun was rising.

I'd set the alarm early to catch the sole bus that day down to Le Bourg-d'Oisans. From there, unless it had been clamped or stolen, I'd drive the car back to where I was staying, Langley Hotel Le Petit Prince, pack up my bike, bags and bits, drive to Lyon Airport and fly home.

While I was waiting for the bus, I got chatting to a local by the name of Benjamin, a former military man who now worked as a maintenance chap in Alpe d'Huez. He was meeting a friend in Le Bourg-d'Oisans. 'You rode up Croix de Fer? Yesterday? In that heat? You crazy man. How old are you? Forty-five? You're not 20, you fool!' After appraising my age and mental state, he guided me to the cafe for an espresso and a solitary pastry. 'This will help you,' he guaranteed. Again, not textbook nutrition but as my stomach felt knotted from the previous day's gastro and race distress, it was good enough.

As it had to be, because after much French and English cursing, the bus never showed up. And with that, Benjamin walked away. This wasn't great. I called a taxi. No answer. I called another taxi. No answer. 'Hmm, my legs don't feel too bad, certainly better than after a marathon,' I pondered to myself. 'I have plenty of time to catch my flight. Hmm.' Sadly, I'd returned the hire front wheel and didn't fancy pulling a wheely 13.8km down a steep mountain.

And so it was I spent the next two and a half hours walking the road that I'd travelled along 12 hours before. This time, though, I was bike-free, in trainers rather than cleats, and downhill not up. As the sun had yet to rise to high, it was also at least 10°C cooler than when I'd started at the foothills of Alpe d'Huez the evening before.

Alpe d'Huez was a place transformed. Where I'd earlier seen fear, now I saw beauty. Pines flanked the roads, leaving a fresh aroma. All I'd been able to smell before was the sunscreen that had streamed into my eyes and down my nose. Alpine flowers added colour while the sound of trickling water made this feel like the healthiest place on Earth. What a difference a day makes. The verges were beginning to fill with fans and tents in preparation for the Pidcock Roadshow to follow in three days' time. And an easy flow of recreational cyclists passed me as they ascended Huez, including two who had Étape race numbers still zip-tied to their bikes. 'Show-offs,' I muttered.

I then noticed the first of what would be 21 signs (in homage to the 21 stages of the Tour de France) celebrating past winners atop Alpe d'Huez, plus the exact altitude at each sign's location. These start with sign number '21' at the base featuring Fausto Coppi, the first to win here in 1952, and finish on the last hairpin with sign '1', featuring Giuseppe Guerini, who won here in 1999. In-between are the winners in chronological order.

The backdrop, the hairpins, the time to play with – all three combined to give me ample opportunity to reflect on the highs and lows of a journey that began all those months ago with a brutal fitness test and ended with an even more brutal race. What's more, walking past the signs bearing the names of the giants of cycling gave this Everyman a chance to contemplate what lessons I could pass on to other Every(wo)men who might consider rising to the same (or a similar) challenge...

1	HAVE A PLAN
♐	*Giuseppe Guerini, Italy, 1999* *1713m*

When it comes to training, you don't necessarily need to be structured. I say that as someone whose consistency of sessions has wavered over the years. Sometimes, like when I ran the London Marathon, I followed a plan. Often, like racing a few triathlons, my training was relatively ad hoc. However, despite my draining display in France, I really enjoyed the structure and variety of the programme I followed this time. Rather neatly, the sessions would sync to my TrainingPeaks calendar and instantly feed back details such as intensity, speed and calories burned. I can't thank Phil Mosley enough for his coaching input, even if I didn't quite manage to make the podium.

2	EMBRACE THE EFFICIENT
♐	*Marco Pantani, Italy, 1997* *1669m*

Once, I was so bored of riding indoors that my nose fell off and I nearly died. Hyperbole, perhaps, but when I first attempted turbo training over 20 years ago, I thought there was little out there that could kill the joy of cycling with such searing dullness. Now, it's a sector of cycling that's been transformed due to the stimulating duo of smart trainers and multiplayer online platforms like Zwift. Smart trainers even connect to your laptop and, rather smartly, the resistance will change depending on the terrain. You can also sync power meter software like TrainingPeaks, which will recreate your sessions in Zwift world. Smart trainers start from a couple of hundred quid while something like the Wattbike is around £50 a month to hire or £1000-plus for certain models. Indoor riding was absolutely vital to me following the training plan as I could just walk downstairs, hop on and away I went. They also enable you to train hot, which, as we've seen, is useful.

3	FOOD ON THE FLY
🚴	*Marco Pantani, Italy, 1995* *1626m*

Whether it was the crisp-fuelled cobbled odyssey or erratic eating at the Étape, planning what food to eat and when shot off my radar the moment I left England. I can apportion the blame to admin (race signing on), transit (healthy food and driving aren't often happy bedfellows) and tiredness (being too knackered to hit a restaurant), but ultimately the finger of nutritional blame points at me. To rectify the situation wouldn't have taken long. A simple search of supermarkets and eateries near to my hotel would have at least given me options to consider. If the field's expected to be large – like the one at the Étape – it's worth booking ahead if that's feasible.

4	REFLECT, TWEAK, REFLECT...
🚴	*Roberto Conti, Italy, 1994* *1553m*

The band of world-class experts who helped shape my position, feeding and training were brilliant. But they can only do so much, and they obviously aren't accessible or affordable for everyone. I can thank Phil Burt for ensuring I didn't once suffer from lower-back pain, knee pain or shoulder pain, which were three major concerns with the increase in mileage. His analysis resulted in a higher, more efficient saddle position, plus he moulded bespoke insoles to help with my clawing toes. Which seemed to do the job. However, a few times on this journey, my right foot quietly flared up before going AWOL at the Étape. I should have contacted Phil when those hints of pain first appeared as he'd have offered a further solution. Experts need their subjects to feed back to optimise their knowledge.

5	**MAINTAINING MOTIVATION**
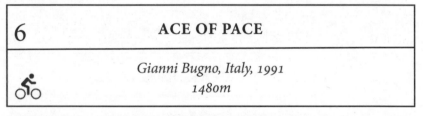	*Andy Hampsten, USA, 1992* *1512m*

I might not have racked up the finishing time I was after but I finished. And there was absolutely no way that would have happened if the motivation hadn't been strong enough, both at the race and in training. New Year's resolutions are easy. The difficult part is making them stick. Hence why so many gym-goers struggle to exercise into February. But as L'Étape du Tour did for me, your challenge must excite you but also be within the realms of possibility. It's why merely pencilling in next year's yellow jersey in my diary might not motivate me to ride – it's simply not attainable.

6	**ACE OF PACE**
	Gianni Bugno, Italy, 1991 *1480m*

Whether it's by heart rate, speed or power, a proficient pacing strategy is a must for a long day in the saddle. Not only will it help you judge efforts that can stretch to, well, 12 hours, but it'll also help you remain in control when the thrill of the race – like the start – can see you ride on emotion … and then bonk as you've overdone it. I'd have been interested to see if my 160–200-watt strategy would have paid off if my stomach hadn't become slightly confused. Next time…

7	**YOU ARE NOT A PRO!**
	Gianni Bugno, Italy, 1990 *1390m*

I'm sounding like a scratched record but while challenges of this nature demand a high level of commitment, this isn't your job, livelihood, everything. Yes, you need to train consistently, progressively, at times intensively, sometimes for many, many hours of the day. It can take over your life. If that suits your life, chapeau to you. But for most of us, this is just part of the picture, not the whole picture. Work, social life, family, parties, weddings, stag-dos … there's a lot to juggle but juggle you must if you want to enjoy a rich, rewarding life. Get your mates on board but try to avoid becoming a biking bore.

8	GOAL-SETTING FOR GOAL-GETTING
⚲	*Gert-Jan Theunisse, the Netherlands, 1989* *1345m*

Great oaks from little acorns grow and all that… Goal setting is the surest way of goal-getting. Yes, that is a rubbish phrase but it's true. If you don't have a clear target, how are you going to reach it? For me, the plan worked wonders, as did the trickle of races, from the cyclo-cross in Keynsham and the time trial in Dursley to the Flanders sportive. They all built towards the bigger goal of the Étape.

There are many psychological models out there that can help you to set your own goals. One favoured by top sports psychologist Josephine Perry is the SCALED UP model. Over to Perry. 'This stands for Specific; Clear, so you're not tempted to change when it gets hard; Achievable; Layered – when we focus only on outcome, we develop unrealistic future expectations and these reduce our confidence, increase anxiety, stop us putting so much effort in and cause poor performance. It's the performance and process goals [of which more to follow] that help us develop more realistic expectations; Exciting; Deadline – sometimes life gets in the way of our sport, deadlines help us stay on track; U – focused as much as possible on things you can control; Positive – focusing on what you're trying to achieve, not on what you want to avoid.'

9	**ALCOHOL-FREE**
🚴	*Steven Rooks, the Netherlands, 1988* *1295m*

Reading back on my roller-coaster of a journey, at times it looks like I'm the new George Best – and sadly I don't mean because of my footballer trickery. I'm not a heavy boozer, 'only' drinking two or three times a week. In itself, though, that's not great as each drink can come in at around 200 calories, so that's around 800 to 1000 calories on Friday and Saturday nights, plus the extra piled on from making rubbish food choices when mildly inebriated. When I was in my 20s and early 30s, I could seemingly manage this without adding a pound. Nowadays, that's not possible. I found two alcohol-free blocks that totalled nine weeks were beneficial, certainly when it came to losing weight, which was needed in this heavily weight-based challenge. Many people would consider quitting alcohol for the duration of their training, and good for them. Then again, life is for living. I didn't quite feel at the stage of not drinking at the stag-do I'd organised, nor at Kempo's wedding. Balance is key but cutting alcohol for even a short while really does help if that's all you feel you can manage.

10	**HIT THE HILLS**
🚴	*Federico Echave, Spain, 1987* *1245m*

This was arguably the biggest thing I'd change if I had my time again. I rode many hills but still not as often as I should have. I've mentioned the Bath to Lansdown climb, which is a beast, and I rode to Cheddar Gorge and back a few times. But in following the plan pretty much verbatim, I made an error. That's because the online plan gave impressive detail, like when to change power and for how long, but it didn't really mention hills. So, while I blindly followed the routine according to intensity, distance and time, that often came at the expense of seeking out gradients. Next time – fanciful! – I'd spend time on VeloViewer to seek out nearby hills and be a little more gradient methodical.

11	SOME NEED TO LIKE IT HOT MORE OFTEN
♂	*Bernard Hinault, France, 1986* *1195m*

I'd visited a heat chamber, endured hot baths and cycled hundreds of miles indoors without airflow to cool me down. All of this I'd hope helped me to acclimatise to the 40°C-plus temperatures on the roads of south-eastern France. However, in retrospect, I felt I should have done more. Even if I'd not suffered from stomach issues in the build-up, that heat would have caused severe problems. You can only do so much to prepare but longer indoor rides with the heating cranked up would have helped. As would losing a few more pounds because higher fitness leads to many adaptations that are conducive to riding in the heat, such as better thermoregulation.

12	THE LONG RIDE
♂	*Luis Herrera, Colombia, 1984* *1161m*

The weekly long ride or run is pretty standard fare for most endurance training programmes and with good reason: it boosts aerobic capacity, helps you to become leaner and biomechanically prepares you for the long race to come. I enjoyed mine until around the four-hour mark. Then, with much on my plate – did I mention we sold our house?! – it felt almost irresponsible to be out so long. It also grew a little boring. That's where riding with others or even joining a club would have helped. I noticed in France especially just how much the shortest of chats could distract the mind from pain and distance, particularly if you come across an amusing bugger like Cillian from GCN. If I ever train for such a mountainous race again, I won't ride solo as much.

13	THAT'S ENTERTAINMENT
🚴	*Peter Winnen, the Netherlands, 1983* *Geraint Thomas, Great Britain, 2018* *1120m*

While I used Zwift, I also followed sessions while being entertained by BBC iPlayer, Netflix, YouTube… An hour soon passes when you're riding to the rather hilarious Tim Key and Daisy May Cooper in *The Witchfinder* or watching *A Sunday In Hell*, the 1976 documentary that stylishly chronicled that year's Paris–Roubaix. I also listened to podcasts and Spotify on many a ride via a pair of Aftershokz bone conduction headphones. Podcast favourites include *The Adam Buxton Podcast*, *The Cycling Podcast*, Bob Mortimer's *Athletico Mince* and a number of series on BBC Sounds. The *Hurricane Tapes*, about boxer Rubin Carter, by Steve Crossman was a particular favourite. Usual caveats about riding with music apply though this is where bone conduction versions help as you can still clearly hear around you.

14	THE MIND MATTERS
🚴	*Beat Breu, Switzerland, 1982* *Thibaut Pinot, France, 2015* *1055m*

I left my session with sports psychologist Noel Brick not only full of confidence but also armed with psychological tricks to ease the pain. Granted, these were tested to the limit when climbing the Alpe d'Huez but I'd certainly tap into the services of a sports psychologist again. Yes, I'd interviewed many over the years, written features about them, but it's only when using one that I realised just how beneficial they can be. Seeking help from a sports nutritionist is also a wise shout, not only if budget allows but also if you're also new to endurance sport.

15	PROTECT YOUR PRIDE AND JOY

Peter Winnen, the Netherlands, 1981
Christophe Riblon, France, 2013
1025m

A good bike box is worth its weight in gold. Cue the Bike Box Alan that a friend kindly lent me. The model in question was the Triathlon Aero Easyfit, which proved particularly useful as I didn't need to break down the bars. It's £635, though, so unless you're constantly riding or racing abroad, you might be better served hiring one. Prices start from around £40. Just remember that whatever box or bag you choose, it can only do so much. Also sort insurance, either standalone or as a top-up.

16	MORE THAN THE BIKE

Joop Zoetemelk, the Netherlands, 1979*
Pierre Rolland, France, 2011
980m

Swathes of carbon, streamlined helmets, deep-rim wheels, tubing that's derived from space shuttle research – the lure of aerodynamic gear is strong. But sort yourself out first. Popular consensus says you are 80 per cent of drag, so positioning, weight and clothing will all help. You don't need to squeeze into a suit spawned from the Vorteq labs but non-flappy clothing is an easy aero win. Remember: at an event like the Étape, you'll be out there much longer than the professionals, so aerodynamics is arguably even more important. But sort yourself out first, then your bike.

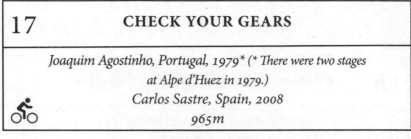

17	**CHECK YOUR GEARS**
	Joaquim Agostinho, Portugal, 1979* (* There were two stages at Alpe d'Huez in 1979.)
	Carlos Sastre, Spain, 2008
	965m

I'd like to think that I would have walked less up Alpe d'Huez if I'd started with a full tank. But I also needed lower gears. When the gradients hit 10%, I really struggled and just didn't have low enough options to climb like a goat. This was an oversight that wouldn't happen again. Your local mechanic will be able to offer good advice on the best gear ratios for your abilities and upcoming parcours.

18	**YOU CAN SPREAD THE LOVE**
	Hennie Kuiper, the Netherlands, 1978
	Frank Schleck, Luxemburg, 2006
	922m

It's common for passionate road cyclists to focus solely on cycling, which is fine – they live it, breathe it, love it. I'm a huge fan of cycling, too, whether it's watching or reporting on the professionals, or riding my road bike. But I also enjoy mountain biking, bikepacking adventures and even commuting. Cycling's a wonderful activity in all forms, of which I enjoy many. But at heart, I simply love sport, both living it vicariously and through participation. It's why I just couldn't give up that five-a-side, even if the risk of injury or muscle damage was high. Road cycling is wonderful, but don't feel you're being disloyal by loving other sports.

19	**SMILE LIKE YOU MEAN IT**
	Hennie Kuiper, the Netherlands, 1977
	Lance Armstrong, USA, 2004
	900m

Smile. Not only does research show that this simple act lessens the pain, but cycling should be enjoyable. Smile and let the good times roll.

20	**PAIN IS PART OF THE PLEASURE**
⚲	*Joop Zoetemelk, the Netherlands, 1976* *Iban Mayo, Spain, 2003* *880m*

'Cyclists live with pain. If you can't handle it, you will win nothing. The race is won by the rider who can suffer the most.' These were the words of Eddy Merckx when he was asked about the relationship between cycling and suffering. Fausto Coppi rolled out an even briefer response: 'Cycling is suffering.' It begs the questions: what is suffering? And if it's such a strong identifier of road cycling, how can we dig deeper to widen our suffering bandwidth and race faster, longer, stronger? Despite the reams of data churned out by power meters and analysed by sophisticated algorithms, we can't objectively measure 'suffering'. But you'll know it when you come across it. And when you do, you'll discover your capabilities are far greater than you'd ever imagined. This will surely hold you in good stead for other facets of your life. Time will tell but I suspect I learned more about myself during 12 hours of hot suffering than at any time in my life. 'Every turn of the wheel, my friend,' as Kempo would say.

21	**ME, ME, ME**
⚲	*Fausto Coppi, Italy, 1952* *Lance Armstrong, USA, 2001* *806m*

I enjoyed great support from family, friends and industry experts. But at the end of the day, I was only really accountable to myself. It was I who would succeed or fail depending on my decisions and my actions. This is something hammered home by the high-performers interviewed by Jake Humphreys and Damian Hughes on their *High Performance* podcast. I'd recommend listening.

Physio Phil Burt also hammered this home early on. 'I remember when Steve Peters came into British Cycling and brought in what he called "Holding the mirror up", he told me. 'A rider would sit with him, telling him their problems and he'd say, "Is that a real problem or is that just you? I think we're focusing on the wrong thing here. The problem isn't your coach or equipment, it's you. You're externalising failure."'

This lack of accountability is a major hurdle to progress; self-awareness is a key trait of successful athletes, as they're generally aware of rate-limiting steps. 'At British Cycling, we had "what it takes to win" plans,' Burt continued. 'On a big whiteboard, you'd state, "What is the goal?" Then this is where we are and this is where we need to get to. How steep is that curve? If you have four weeks and need to add another 150 watts, it isn't going to happen. So, goals must be achievable but challenging.'

I reached the base of Alpe d'Huez tired, dehydrated but buoyant after such a memorable – and fraught – weekend. The car wasn't clamped, I made it to Lyon Airport, the flight was on time and I arrived back in Bristol safe and sound. It had been a memorable year, filled with the highs of Andorran air, the lows of bike thievery and many cobbled, aerodynamic and weight-shedding memories in-between. Unlike Steve Redgrave and his banishing boat comment, I did want to see another bike again. It's the most beautiful activity that's there for your every need. From short commutes to long days in the saddle, many of life's environmental, physical and mental challenges are if not conquered, at least helped by this most wonderful of inventions. Right, I'm off for a pint of Clear Head and the next adventure...

REFERENCES

All online resources accessed November 2022.

CHAPTER 1

1. Gallo, G., Mateo-March, M., Gotti, D., Faelli, E., Ruggeri, P., Codella, R. and Filipas, L., 'How do world-class top-5 Giro d'Italia finishers train?', *Scandinavian Journal of Medicine & Science in Sports*, 00 (2022), pp. 1–9.
2. *The Economist* magazine, Pedro Zaragoza Orts obituary (April 2008).
3. Nagle, K. B. and Brooks, A. B., 'A Systematic Review of Bone Health in Cyclists', *Sports Health*, 3(3) (2011), pp. 235–243.

CHAPTER 3

4. Carmichael, R. D., Heikkinen, D. J., Mullin, E. M. and McCall, N. R., 'Physiological response to cyclo-cross racing', *Sports and Exercise Medicine*, 3(2) (2017), pp. 74–80.

CHAPTER 4

5. San-Millán, I., Stefanoni, D., Martinez, J. L., Hansen, K. C., D'Alessandro, A. and Nemkov, T., 'Metabolomics of Endurance Capacity in World Tour Professional Cyclists', *Frontiers in Physiology*, doi.org/10.3389/fphys.2020.00578
6. Cooper, C., *Run, Swim, Throw, Cheat: The Science Behind Drugs in Sport* (Oxford University Press 2013).
7. *Combatting doping in sport*, Digital, Culture, Media and Sport Committee (2018), Fourth Report Session of 2017–2019.
8. Hurst, P., Ring, C. and Kavussanu, M., 'Moral values and moral identity moderate the indirect relationship between sport supplement use and doping use via sport supplement beliefs', *Journal of Sports Sciences*, 40 (10) (2022), pp. 1160–1167.
9. Thevis, M., Maurer, J., Kohler, M., Geyer, H. and Schanzer, W., 'Proteases in doping control analysis', *International Journal of Sports Medicine*, 28(7) (2007), pp. 545–549.

CHAPTER 6

10. Bagherian, S. and Rahnama, N., 'Epidemiology of injury in professional cyclists', *British Journal of Sports Medicine*, 44 (2010), p. i4.

11. Haeberle, H. S., Navarro, S. M., Power, E. J., Schickendantz, M. S., Farrow, L. D. and Ramkumar, P. N., 'Prevalence and epidemiology of injuries among elite cyclists in the Tour de France', *Orthopaedic Journal of Sports Medicine*, 6(9) (2018).

12. Thomas, K., Stone, M. R., Thompson, K. G., St Clair Gibson, A. and Ansey, L., 'The effect of self-, even- and variable-pacing strategies on the physiological and perceptual response to cycling', *European Journal of Applied Physiology*, 112(8) (2012), pp. 3069–3078.

13. Thomas, K., Stone, M., St Clair Gibson, A., Thompson, K. and Ansey, L., 'The effect of an even pacing strategy on exercise tolerance in well-trained cyclists', *European Journal of Applied Physiology*, 113(12) (2013), doi: 10.1007/s00421-013-2734-4.

14. Jeffries, O., Waldron, M., Patterson, S. D. and Galna, B., 'An analysis of variability in power output during indoor and outdoor cycling time trials', *International Journal of Sports Physiology and Performance*, Aug 29 (2019): pp. 1273–1279.

15. Noakes T. D., '1996 J.B. Wolffe memorial lecture. Challenging beliefs: ex-Africa semper aliquid novi', *Medicine & Science in Sports & Exercise*, 29(5) (1997), pp. 571–590.

CHAPTER 7

16. Rodriguez-Marroyo, J. A., Villa, J. G., Pernia, R. and Foster, C., 'Decrement in professional cyclists' performance after a Grand Tour', *International Journal of Sports Physiology and Performance,* 12(10) (2017), pp. 1348–1355.

17. Bellenger, C. R., Miller, D. J., Halson, S. L., Roach, G. D. and Sargent, C., 'Wrist-based photoplethysmography assessment of heart rate and heart rate variability: validation of Whoop', *Sensors*, 21(10) (May 2021), p. 3571.

18. Freeman, R., *The Line: Where Medicine and Sport Collide* (Wildfire Publishing 2018).

19. Lowry, A., '10-year journey: Chris Froome on dropping out of university to conquer the cycling world', *Shortlist* magazine (2017).

20. Schmid, S. M., Hallschmid, M., Jauch-Chara, K., Born, J. and Schultes, B., 'A single night of sleep deprivation increases ghrelin levels and feelings of hunger in normal-weight healthy men', *Journal of Sleep Research*, 17(3) (2008): pp. 331–334.

21. Center for Environmental Therapeutics, Morningness-Eveningness Questionnaire. Available at: https://chronotype-self-test.info/index .php?sid=61524&newtest=Y

CHAPTER 8

22. Jeukendrup, A., 'Nutrition during a Grand Tour'. Available at: www .mysportscienceacademy.com/course/nutrition-during-a-grand-tour (2022)

23. Volpi, E., Nazemi, R. and Fujita, S., 'Muscle tissue changes with aging', *Current Opinion in Clinical Nutrition & Metabolic Care*, 7(4) (July 2004), pp. 405–410.

24. Bailey, S. J., Winyard, P., Vanhatalo, A., Blackwell, J. R., Dimenna, F. J., Wilkerson, D. P., Tarr, J., Benjamin, N. and Jones, A. M., 'Dietary supplementation reduces the O2 cost of low-intensity exercise and enhances tolerance to high-intensity exercise in humans', *Journal of Applied Physiology*, 107(4) (October 2009), pp. 1144–1155.

CHAPTER 9

25. Mateo-March, M., Mureil, X., Valenzuela, P. L., Gandia-Soriano, A., Zabala, M., Barranco-Gil, D., Pallares, J. G. and Lucia, A., 'Altitude and endurance performance in altitude natives versus lowlanders: insights from professional cycling', *Medicine & Science in Sports & Exercise*, 54(7) (July 2022), pp. 1218–1224.

26. *Chris Boardman: The Final Hour*, YouTube. Available at: www.youtube .com/watch?v=kWdwSOX6B0A

27. Lee, B. J., Miller, A., James, R. S. and Charles, D., 'Cross acclimation between heat and hypoxia: heat acclimation improves cellular tolerance and exercise performance in acute normobaric hypoxia', *Frontiers in Physiology*, doi: https://doi.org/10.3389/fphys.2016.00078

28. Zurawlew, M. J., Walsh, N. P., Fortes, M. B. and Potter C., 'Post-exercise hot water immersion induces heat acclimation and improves endurance exercise performance in the heat', *Scandinavian Journal of*

Medicine & Science in Sports, (205), doi: https://doi.org/10.1111/sms
.12638

CHAPTER 10

29. Jones, M. V., Meijen, C., McCarthy, P. J. and Sheffield, D., 'A theory of challenge and threat states in athletes', *International Review of Sport and Exercise Psychology*, 2 (2009), pp. 161–180.

ACKNOWLEDGEMENTS

First of all, the fine team at Bloomsbury, especially Megan Jones whose iron fist in a velvet glove ensured a finer end product while I (nearly) hit my deadlines.

My agent, Kevin Pocklington, who justified his generous cut. We're forever bonded by 'that' Rouleur Classic moment.

My good friend and prolific author Nige Tassell, who proved vital in fleshing out the idea and title. I owe you a veg pasty at our next Hellenic league match.

All the teams and experts who were so generous with their time and guidance. Special thanks go to the human bullet that is Dan Bigham of Ineos Grenadiers for organising access to Andorra; Phil Mosley, a wonderful coach; the team at Wiggle for the loan of the Vitus; Phil Burt, the burly Cornishman who laid the foundations for my journey; the team at Vorteq; Laurence Gauthier of ASO, who sorted me an Etape media place – I cursed you every step up Alpe d'Huez; and the genius who offered peaches on the final food stop in Bourg d'Oisans.

My good friends Ian 'Now Little Man Due To His Continued Obsession With Zwift' Kemp and Timbo Jackson for their continued support and collective cobble wobble of Flanders. Bikes and beer in Belgium will remain long in the memory.

My mum and dad who taught me to ride a bike ... and then picked me up and cleaned me up when I flew off after my paperbag got caught in the front wheel. Hopefully, my father will enjoy this as much as my first book, *The Science of the Tour de France*, where he regularly phoned me to tell me how much he was enjoying the start of chapter one. You are both the best.

My sister Lou, who's a constant pillar of support. You may have a pinhead but you have a heart of gold.

My children, Mia and Harold, who generously put up with pools of Wattbike-stimulated sweat while cooking lunch. You delight and challenge in equal measure!

And finally, my wife, best friend and the lady who insists on being called 'err indoors', Tara. My Étape challenge was nothing compared to your battle with long Covid. You are amazing, beautiful ... and unique.

APPENDIX 1: TRAINING NOTES

The journey to hell takes many forms…

[Disclaimer: Training notes are not be followed as professional advice etc.]

24-week training plan for James Witts up to Sunday, 10 July 2022

Monday 24 January
60-min five-a-side football

Wednesday 26 January
Strength and conditioning (S&C)

Whole body strength:
1 Squat: 2 x 12
2 Alternate lunge: 2 x 8
3 Single-leg squat: 2 x 6
4 Reverse lunge: 2 x 6
5 Bent-over row: 2 x 12
6 Push-up: 2 x 12
7 Glute bridge: 2 x 12
8 Bird dog: 2 x 7
9 Plank: 1 x 2
10 Reverse crunch: 2 x 12

Flexibility: 5–10 mins.

Notes:
1 2 x 12 = 2 sets of 12 repetitions with a rest between sets.
2 Rests are 20–40 secs.

3 When an exercise alternates right and left, the right PLUS left movement is 1 rep.
4 For unilateral exercises, perform reps on the right, then repeat on the left. Then move to the next set.
5 Breathe out on exertion and maintain form throughout.

Prep phase:
The goal of the prep phase is to develop neuromuscular efficiency, stability and functional strength.

Resistance during the prep phase:
Fairly light weights to enable you to adopt and maintain correct form throughout. If your muscles burn at the end of a set then you are lifting too heavy for this phase.

Perform strength and conditioning once or twice each week. Avoid the 'no pain, no gain' thinking. Strength will complement your training, making you more powerful, less prone to injury and help you focus on a range of movement required for cycling. It should not inhibit your subsequent workouts.

Thursday 27 January
36-min indoor M.A.P. effort session.
M.A.P. stands for Maximal Aerobic Power. It refers to the power output you can ride while at your maximal rate of oxygen consumption. These workouts include efforts that are at or just below your M.A.P.

Warm-up:
7 mins in Z2
5 x (10 secs in Z5 + 50 secs in low Z2)
3 mins in Z2

Main set:
4 x (2 mins in Z5 + 2-min recoveries in low Z2)

Cool-down:
5 mins in low Z2

Phil's training tip:

Don't panic if you cannot complete 100 per cent of your workouts. Do your best to stick to your plan, while accepting that occasionally life gets in the way. Following a plan will help you train more effectively than not having a plan at all. Do your best with whatever time and resources you have, and don't give up. Don't worry about one bad week; it's what you do consistently over a period of months that counts.

Friday 28 January
Easy commuting ride

Sunday 30 January
Cyclo-cross 60 mins

Tuesday 1 February
41-min indoor strength session

Warm-up:
10 mins in Z2
5 x (15 secs in upper Z3 + 45 secs in low Z2)

Main set:
6, 5 and 4 mins in upper Z3 at 60–70rpm + 2-min recoveries in low Z2 at 80–100rpm

Cool-down:
5 mins in low Z2

Phil's comment:
Think of this like a bike-specific gym strength workout. It will increase cycling-related leg-strength, which will help you get more power out of each pedal stroke. Do the warm-up and cool-down at your normal cadence.

Thursday 3 February
38-min indoor M.A.P. effort session

Warm-up:
7 mins in Z2

5 x (10 secs in Z5 + 50 secs in low Z2)
3 mins in Z2

Main set:
2 mins in Z5 + 3 mins' recovery in low Z2
3 mins in Z5 + 3 mins' recovery in low Z2
4 mins in Z5 + 3 mins' recovery in low Z2

Cool-down:
5 mins in low Z2

Friday 4 February
1.07.02 outdoor endurance ride
18.3 miles

Sunday 6 February
1.54.57 outdoor endurance ride
23.8 miles

Ride at an easy/steady intensity, mainly in Z2 today. You should be able to chat at this intensity. This ride will improve your efficiency for using fat for fuel and increase your ability to transport oxygen to your working muscles.

Monday 7 February
60-min five-a-side football

Tuesday 8 February
40 mins' S&C

Whole-body strength:
1 Squat: 2 x 12
2 Alternate lunge: 2 x 8
3 Singl-leg squat: 2 x 6
4 Reverse lunge: 2 x 6
5 Bent-over row: 2 x 12
6 Push-up: 2 x 12

7 Glute bridge: 2 x 12
8 Bird dog: 2 x 7
9 Plank: 1 x 2
10 Reverse crunch: 2 x 12

Flexibility: 5–10 mins.

Wednesday 9 February
41-min indoor sub-threshold, low-cadence effort session

Warm-up:
5 mins in Z2
5 x (15 secs in upper Z3 + 45 secs in low Z2)

Main set:
2 x (10 mins in upper Z3 at 60–70rpm + 3-min recoveries in low Z2
at 80–100rpm)

Cool-down:
5 mins in low Z2

Also, two 20-min commuting rides to Bristol and back

Friday 11 February
57-min indoor endurance ride
Plus 55 mins of commuting

Sunday 13 February
2.01.44 outdoor endurance ride
First Lansdown ride. That hill is tough. Damn cold feet. Mainly Z2
but hit maximum of 170bpm when climbing to Lansdown.

Tuesday 15 February
1.02.00 indoor endurance ride

Warm-up:
10 mins in Z2
5 x (20 secs in Z3 + 40 secs in low Z2)

Main set:
3 x (8 mins in upper Z2 + 30-sec recoveries in low Z2)
3 x (5 mins in upper Z2 + 30-sec recoveries in low Z2)

Cool-down:
5 mins in low Z2

Tuesday 15 February
1.02.00 indoor endurance ride

Warm-up:
10 mins in Z2
5 x (20 secs in Z3 + 40 secs in low Z2)

Main set:
3 x (8 mins in upper Z2 + 30-sec recoveries in low Z2)
3 x (5 mins in upper Z2 + 30-sec recoveries in low Z2)

Cool-down:
5 mins in low Z2

Thursday 17 February
37-min indoor M.A.P. effort session

Warm-up:
10 mins in Z2
5 x (10 secs in Z5 + 50 secs in low Z2)
3 mins in Z2

Main set:
2 x (4 mins in Z5 + 3-min recoveries in low Z2)

Cool-down:
5 mins in low Z2

Friday 18 February
1.02.43 indoor Zwift aerobic effort session
Instead of Sunday ride as heading to Lisbon with chubhead (my son, Harry)

Sunday 20 February
37-min indoor ride
At Lisbon gym. Parochial set-up

Monday 21 February
10km run
Interval training set as sprinting around Lisbon with the Portuguese running tour guide

Tuesday 22 February
40 mins' S&C

Whole-body strength:
1 Squat: 3 x 12
2 Single-leg squat: 3 x 8
3 Bulgarian squat: 3 x 10
4 Bench press: 3 x 10
5 Tricep kickback: 3 x 10
6 Bent-over row: 3 x 10
7 Mountain climber: 3 x 8
8 Reverse crunch: 3 x 12
9 Plank: 1 x 3

Wednesday 23 February
53.14-min indoor endurance ride

Friday 25 February
1.04.00 indoor endurance ride

Warm-up:
10 mins in Z2
5 x (20 secs in Z3 + 40 secs in low Z2)

Main set:
4 x (10 mins in upper Z2 + 60-sec recoveries in low Z2)

Cool-down:
5 mins in low Z2

Sunday 27 February
2.08.44 outdoor endurance ride
27.2 miles

Ride mainly in Z2 today. You should be able to maintain conversation at this intensity.

Monday 28 February
60-min five-a-side football

Wednesday 2 March
41-min indoor threshold effort session

Warm-up:
10 mins in low Z2
5 x (10 secs in Z4 + 50 secs in low Z2)

Main set:
4 x (2 mins in upper Z4 + 2-min recoveries in low Z2)

Cool-down:
5 mins in upper Z2
5 mins in low Z2

Plus two commuting rides of 22.30 mins

Thursday 3 March
40-min indoor M.A.P effort session

Warm-up:
8 mins in Z2
5 x (10 secs in Z5 + 50 secs in low Z2)
2 mins in Z2

Main set:
20 x (30 secs in Z5 + 30 secs in low Z2)

Cool-down:
5 mins in low Z2

Friday 4 March
22-min commuting ride

Saturday 5 March
54-min indoor endurance ride

Warm-up:
10 mins in Z2
5 x (30 secs in upper Z2 + 30 secs in low Z2)

Main set:
9 mins in upper Z2 + 60-sec recovery in low Z2
7 mins in upper Z2 + 60-sec recovery in low Z2
5 mins in upper Z2 + 60-sec recovery in low Z2
3 mins in upper Z2 + 60-sec recovery in low Z2
1 min in upper Z2

Cool-down:
10 mins in mid Z2

Sunday 6 March
2.10.00 outdoor endurance ride
Indoors as freezing!

Monday 7 March
60-min five-a-side football, plus two 40-min rides to football and back

Tuesday 8 March
25-min commuting ride

Wednesday 9 March
41-min indoor M.A.P. effort session

Warm-up:
7 mins in Z2
5 x (10 secs in Z5 + 50 secs in low Z2)
3 mins in Z2

Main set:
7 x (90 secs in Z5 + 90-sec recoveries in low Z2)

Cool-down:
5 mins in low Z2

Thursday 10 March
27-min commute ride
Felt tired

Saturday 12 March
57-min outdoor endurance ride
16 miles

Sunday 13 March
2.30.00 outdoor endurance ride.
A jaunt from Bristol to past Clevedon and back. Stopped to see if any houses are for sale!

Monday 14 March
60-min five-a-side football

Wednesday 16 March
1.32.52 outdoor endurance ride.
Another ride from Bristol to past Clevedon and back.

Thursday 17 March
36-min indoor M.A.P. effort session

Warm-up:
7 mins in Z2
5 x (10 secs in Z5 + 50 secs in low Z2)
3 mins in Z2

Main set:
4 x (2 mins in Z5 + 2-min recoveries in low Z2)

Cool-down:
5 mins in low Z2

Friday 18 March
28-min indoor ride
Have a heavy cold so will miss long ride on the Sunday

Monday 21 March
60-min five-a-side football

Tuesday 22 March
50-min fitness test
This fitness test helps you update your power and heart rate thresholds
for TrainingPeaks

Warm-up:
15 mins in Z2
5 mins as (15 secs in Z4 + 45 secs easy in Z2)

Main set:
20 mins maximal steady state time trial. Go as hard as you can sustain
for 20 mins

Cool-down:
10 mins in Z2

Plus two 20-min commuting rides

Thursday 24 March
44-min indoor ride
Newcastle for son's university open day. Recovering from cold.
Muscular tiredness in legs from last few days. On hotel bike. But
workout roughly completed.

Friday 25 March
40-min S&C session
In Newcastle hotel gym

Whole-body strength:
1 Squat: 3 x 16 (Exercise 1)
2 Squat jump: 3 x 8 (Exercise 2)
3 Step-up: 3 x 9 (Exercise 7)
4 Single-leg squat: 3 x 8 (Exercise 3)
5 Push-up: 3 x 12 (Exercise 12)
6 Lat & front raise combo: 3 x 7 (Exercise 10)
7 Glute bridge: 3 x 14 (Exercise 16)
8 Lying hip abduction: 3 x 12 (Exercise 18)
9 Reverse crunch: 3 x 14 (Exercise 26)

Flexibility: 5–10 mins

Saturday 26 March

2.40.00 outdoor endurance ride.
Cycle from Bristol to the glory that is Weston-super-Mare and back

Monday 28 March

60-min five-a-side football. Felt very tired.

Tuesday 29 March

48-min indoor sub-threshold, low-cadence effort session

Warm-up:
5 mins in Z2
5 x (15 secs in upper Z3 + 45 secs in low Z2)

Main set:
11, 9 and 7 mins in upper Z3 at 60–70rpm + 2 mins' recovery in low
Z2 at 80–100rpm

Cool-down:
5 mins in low Z2

Thursday 31 March

28-min indoor ride
Easy session as Flanders on Saturday

Saturday 2 April, Tour of Flanders Sportive

6.29.24 (7.29.31 with fuel stops!) 90 miles including 2000m climbing

Thursday 7 April

56-min indoor ride
First ride since Flanders after cough

Friday 8 April

40-min indoor ride
Again, easy as cough. This week saw a few commuting rides but recovering from Flanders.

Friday 15 April

35-min indoor M.A.P effort session

Warm-up:
10 mins in Z2
5 x (10 secs in Z5 + 50 secs in low Z2)
3 mins in Z2

Main set:
3 x (2 mins in Z5 + 2-min recoveries in low Z2)

Cool-down:
5 mins in low Z2

Saturday 16 April

41-min indoor threshold effort session

Warm-up:
10 mins in low Z2
5 x (10 secs in Z4 + 50 secs in low Z2)

Main set:
7 x (1 min in upper Z4 + 2-min recoveries in low Z2)

Cool-down:
5 mins in low Z2

Sunday 17 April

1.34.25 outdoor endurance ride

Notes from Phil: Be patient, physiological improvements only happen in a 'drip drip' way like coffee pouring through a filter. There are no shortcuts. Whitby and the hill at Sandsend!

Monday 18 April

S&C on holiday in Whitby

Legs and core strength:

1 Squat: 3 x 10
2 Squat jump: 3 x 12
3 Single-leg squat: 3 x 10
4 Step-up: 3 x 12
5 Box jump: 3 x 8
6 Bicycle crunch: 4 x 10
7 Plank: 1 x 3
8 Spider climber: 3 x 10
9 Side plank: 1 x 3

Tuesday 19 April

55-min outdoor threshold effort session on sunny day in Whitby

Warm-up:
10 mins in low Z2
5 x (10 secs in Z4 + 50 secs in low Z2)

Main set:
10 x (1 min in upper Z4 + 2-min recoveries in low Z2)

Cool-down:
5 mins in upper Z2
5 mins in low Z2

Wednesday 20 April

55-min outdoor hill session in Whitby

Friday 22 April

48-min indoor M.A.P. effort session

Warm-up:
7 mins in Z2
5 x (10 secs in Z5 + 50 secs in low Z2)
3 mins in Z2

Main set:
4 x (4 mins in Z5 + 3-min recoveries in low Z2)

Cool-down:
5 mins in low Z2

Sunday 24 April

1.30.00 outdoor endurance ride
Supposed to be 3.30.00 endurance ride but rammed with work and house, and couldn't afford the time – or energy.

Monday 25 April

60-min five-a-side football

Tuesday 26 April

1.08.23 indoor threshold effort session

Warm-up:
10 mins in low Z2
5 x (10 secs in Z4 + 50 secs in low Z2)

Main set:
5 x (2 mins in upper Z4 + 2-min recoveries in low Z2)

Cool-down:
10 mins in upper Z2
5 mins in low Z2

Thursday 28 April

48-min indoor M.A.P. effort session

Warm-up:
7 mins in Z2

5 x (10 secs in Z5 + 50 secs in low Z2)
3 mins in Z2

Main set:
4 x (4 mins in Z5 + 3-min recoveries in low Z2)

Cool-down:
5 mins in low Z2

Saturday 30 April
1.05.00 beach run
On stag weekend in San Sebastian. Little training! Not back until late on Tuesday 3 May.

Thursday 5 May
50-min indoor M.A.P. effort session

Warm-up:
7 mins in Z2
5 x (10 secs in Z5 + 50 secs in low Z2)
3 mins in Z2

Main set:
3 x (3 mins in Z5 + 3-min recoveries in low Z2)
3 x (2 mins in Z5 + 2-min recoveries in low Z2)

Cool-down:
5 mins in low Z2
Felt surprisingly good considering my stomach was still packed with *pintxo* and *cerveza*.

Friday 6 May
1 hr indoor sub-threshold effort session

Warm-up:
20 mins in Z2

Main set:
30 mins in Z2

Cool-down:
10 mins in low Z2

Saturday 7 May
3.54.51 outdoor endurance ride
Longest training ride yet. Beautiful day. Rode past Malmesbury and back. Practised feeding off one gel every 30 mins. Worked well. Electrolyte drinks. Listened to football. Well, started to. Bristol Rovers had to achieve the unthinkable to gain promotion to League One ... and they managed it, beating an already relegated and young Scunthorpe side 7–0. Good day.

Monday 9 May
60-min five-a-side football

Tuesday 10 May
1.1.00 outdoor endurance ride

Thursday 12 May
50-min fitness test

Warm-up:
15 mins in Z2
5 mins as (15 secs in Z4 + 45 secs easy in Z2)

Main set:
20 mins' maximal steady state time trial. Go as hard as you can sustain for 20 mins.

Cool-down:
10 mins in Z2

Plus two 20-min commuting rides

Friday 13 May
45-min indoor ride
Felt tired from test

Sunday 15 May
1.30.00 outdoor endurance ride.
Ride from outskirts of Bristol to Bath and back
Nice and easy in Z2

Monday 16 May
60-min five-a-side football

Tuesday 17 May
20-min commuting ride

Wednesday 18 May
55-min indoor sub-threshold effort session

Warm-up:
10 mins in low Z2
5 x (15 secs in Z4 + 45 secs in low Z2)

Main set:
6 x (3 mins in upper Z4 + 2-min recoveries in low Z2)

Cool-down:
5 mins in upper Z2
5 mins in low Z2

Friday 20 May
50-min indoor ride

Saturday 21 May
3.41.23 outdoor endurance ride
Ride past Chew Valley. Stunning day. Huge waft of wild garlic. Late in the day for such aroma?

Sunday 22 May
Was supposed to ride but felt knackered so rest day

Monday 23 May
60-min five-a-side football

Wednesday 25 May
55-min indoor above and below threshold effort session

Warm-up:
10 mins in low Z2
5 x (10 secs in Z4 + 50 secs in low Z2)

Main set:
10 x (2 mins in Z3 + 30 secs in Z5 + 1 min in low Z2)

Cool-down:
5 mins in low Z2

Thursday 26 May
30 mins' easy indoor ride

Friday 27 May
Kempo's wedding

Saturday 28 May
1.20.00 sub-threshold effort session

Warm-up:
15 mins in Z2

Main set:
4 x (10 mins in upper Z3 + 5-min recoveries in Z2)

Cool-down:
5 mins in low Z2

Sunday 29 May
1 hr outdoor endurance ride
Was supposed to be a 4.20.00 ride but felt fatigued after wedding

Monday 30 May
60-min five-a-side football

Wednesday 1 June
1.00.00 indoor threshold effort session

Warm-up:
10 mins in low Z2
5 x (15 secs in Z4 + 45 secs in low Z2)

Main set:
2 x (10 mins in upper Z4 + 5-min recoveries in low Z2)

Cool-down:
5 mins in upper Z2
10 mins in low Z2

Friday 3 June
4.30.00 outdoor endurance ride
Rode up Cheddar Gorge. Felt OK but mentally a little battered.

Saturday 4 June
1.20.00 outdoor sub-threshold effort session
Ride to Bath and back. Knackered but perked up by Rob Brydon on *Off Menu* with Ed Gamble and James Acaster.

Monday 6 June
60-min five-a-side football

Wednesday 8 June
40-min indoor M.A.P effort session

Warm-up:
10 mins in Z2
5 x (10 secs in Z5 + 50 secs in low Z2)
3 mins in Z2

Main set:
2 x (3 mins in Z5 + 4-min recoveries in low Z2)

Cool-down:
8 mins in low Z2

Thursday 9 June
1.02.00 indoor endurance ride

Warm-up:
7 mins in Z2
5 x (30 secs in upper Z2 + 30 secs in low Z2)

Main set:
16 mins in upper Z2 + 90 secs' recovery in low Z2
14 mins in upper Z2 + 90 secs' recovery in low Z2
12 mins in upper Z2

Cool-down:
5 mins in low Z2

Saturday 11 June
40-min indoor threshold effort session

Warm-up:
10 mins in low Z2
5 x (15 secs in Z4 + 45 secs in low Z2)

Main set:
3 x (3 mins in upper Z4 + 2-min recoveries in low Z2)

Cool-down:
5 mins in upper Z2
5 mins in low Z2

Sunday 12 June
2.00.00 outdoor endurance ride
Lansdown ride. Hoorah – felt much stronger than last time ridden.
Higher cadence, too. Not drinking has done no harm!

Monday 13 June
60-min five-a-side football

Wednesday 15 June
57-min indoor ride

Saturday 18 June
1.35.00 indoor sub-threshold effort session

Warm-up:
15 mins in Z2

Main set:
5 x (10 mins in upper Z3 + 5-min recoveries in Z2)

Cool-down:
5 mins in low Z2

Sunday 19 June
56-min indoor M.A.P. effort session

Warm-up:
7 mins in Z2
5 x (10 secs in Z5 + 50 secs in low Z2)
3 mins in Z2

Main set:
6 x (3 mins in Z5 + 3-min recoveries in low Z2)

Cool-down:
5 mins in low Z2

Note: felt very tired

Monday 20 June
Two 35-min sessions
Fitness test at Porsche plus heat session. Hence, not too much the week before.

Tuesday 21 June
30-min commuting ride

Wednesday 22 June
54-min indoor threshold effort session

Warm-up:
10 mins in low Z2
5 x (15 secs in Z4 + 45 secs in low Z2)

Main set:
4 x (3 mins in upper Z4 + 90-sec recoveries in low Z2)
2 mins 30 secs of extra recovery in low Z2
3 x (3 mins in upper Z4 + 90-sec recoveries in low Z2)

Cool-down:
5 mins in low Z2

Friday 24 June
56-min indoor M.A.P effort session

Warm-up:
7 mins in Z2
5 x (10 secs in Z5 + 50 secs in low Z2)
3 mins in Z2

Main set:
9 x (2 mins in Z5 + 2-min recoveries in low Z2)

Cool-down:
5 mins in low Z2

Saturday 25 June
1.08.07 indoor ride

Sunday 26 June
4.50.00 outdoor endurance ride
Cheddar Gorge and deep into Mendips. Felt good.

Tuesday 28 June
50-min indoor threshold effort session

Warm-up:
10 mins in low Z2
5 x (15 secs in Z4 + 45 secs in low Z2)

Main set:
6 mins in upper Z4 + 3 mins' recovery in low Z2
7 mins in upper Z4 + 3 mins' recovery in low Z2
8 mins in upper Z4 + 3 mins' recovery in low Z2

Cool-down:
5 mins in low Z2

Thursday 30 June
48-min indoor M.A.P. effort session

Warm-up:
7 mins in Z2
5 x (10 secs in Z5 + 50 secs in low Z2)
3 mins in Z2

Main set:
3 x (5 mins in Z5 + 4-min recoveries in low Z2)

Cool-down:
6 mins in low Z2

Saturday 2 July
1.15.00 indoor sub-threshold effort session

Warm-up:
20 mins in Z2

Main set:
3 x (10 mins in upper Z3 + 5 mins' recovery in Z2)

Cool-down:
10 mins in low Z2

Sunday 3 July
4 hr outdoor endurance ride
Last lone ride before L'Étape du Tour. Felt a little throaty!

Wednesday 6 July
1.02.25 easy indoor ride

Friday 8 July
35-min indoor M.A.P. effort session
Last lone ride

Warm-up:
7 mins in Z2
5 x (10 secs in Z5 + 50 secs in low Z2)
3 mins in Z2

Main set:
3 x (2 mins in Z5 + 3-min recoveries in low Z2)

Cool-down:
5 mins in low Z2

Sunday 10 July, L'Étape du Tour
Whisker under 12 hrs. 169km and 4614m of ascent. Average heart rate of 140bpm and max of 171bpm

APPENDIX 2: PRO RIDER'S
RACE CALENDAR

Name: Thomas Pidcock
DOB: 30 July 1999
Nationality: British
Team: Ineos Grenadiers
Height: 1.7m
Weight: 58kg

Cyclo-cross 2021/2022

1 January	X2o Trofee Baal – GP Sven Nys, Baal, Belgium, 2nd
2 January	UCI World Cup Hulst, the Netherlands, 1st
4 January	Hexia Cyclocross Gullegem, Belgium, 1st
5 January	X2o Trofee Herentals, Belgium, 2nd
22 January	X2o Trofee Hamme – Flandriencross, Belgium, 5th
23 January	UCI World Cup Hoogerheide, the Netherlands, 3rd
30 January	UCI World Championships, USA, 1st

Road season 2022

16–20 February	Volta ao Algarve, Portugal, 798.1km. Completed four stages but DNF in fifth and final stage
26 February	Omloop Het Nieuwsblad, 204.2km. Ghent to Ninove, Belgium, 18th
27 February	Kuurne–Brussels–Kuurne, 195.1km. Kuurne to Kuurne, Belgium, 70th
19 March	Milan–Sanremo, 293km. Milan to San Remo, Italy, DNF
27 March	Gent–Wevelgem, 248.8km. Ypres to Wevelgem, Belgium, 67th
30 March	Dwars door Vlaanderen, 183.7km. Roeselare to Wevelgem, Belgium, 3rd
3 April	Tour of Flanders, 272.5km. Antwerp to Oudenaarde, Belgium, 14th

10 April	Amstel Gold Race, 254.1km. Maastricht to Valkenburg, Belgium, 11th
13 April	De Brabantse Pijl, 205.1km. Leuven to Overijse, Belgium, 5th
20 April	La Flèche Wallonne, 202.1km. Blegny to Mur de Huy, Belgium, DNF
24 April	Liège–Bastogne–Liège, 257.2km. Liège to Liège, Belgium, 103rd
12–19 June	Tour de Suisse, 1339.6km. Completed five stages, including a fourth and fifth, but didn't start for stage six
1–24 July	Tour de France, 3238km. 16th overall including victory on stage 12 from Briançon to Alpe d'Huez
4–8 September	Tour of Britain. 2nd overall

Cyclo-cross 2022/2023

19 November	Superprestige Merksplas, Belgium, 7th
20 November	UCI World Cup Overijse, Belgium, 2nd
26 November	X2O Trofee Kortrijk – Urban Cross, Belgium, 1st
27 November	UCI World Cup Hulst, Netherlands, DNF
3 December	Superprestige Boom, Belgium, 1st
4 December	UCI World Cup Antwerp, Belgium, 8th Pidcock also races mountain bike and won gold at the 2020 Tokyo Olympics…

MTB season 2022

6 May	Mercedes-Benz UCI MTB World Cup, cross-country short, Germany, 8th
8 May	Mercedes-Benz UCI MTB World Cup, cross-country Olympic, Germany, 1st
13 May	Mercedes-Benz UCI MTB World Cup, cross-country short, Czech Republic, 2nd
15 May	Mercedes-Benz UCI MTB World Cup, cross-country Olympic, Czech Republic, 1st
19 August	European Continental Championships, cross-country Olympic, Germany, 1st
19 August	UCI MTB World Championships, cross-country Olympic, France, 4th